Praise for Power through Collaboration

"Predatory capitalism took the reins in the 1970s; its emphasis on selfish, often ruthless profit maximization without regard for social and environmental costs led us to the brink of global systemic collapse. Stephen Willis's trailblazing book guides us along a path to the type of collaboration that can pull us back from the precipice - something that is needed as never before!"

John Perkins, New York Times bestselling author of Confessions of an Economic Hit Man, Hoodwinked, Shapeshifting, and many other books that have sold over 1 million copies in 30 languages. He was chief economist of an international consulting firm and advised heads of state and Fortune 500 CEOs, and currently lectures at conferences around the world.

"I am glad to have such a helpful book in my win-win toolkit. And I recommend that it be in the strategic arsenal of not only practitioners, but also business leaders in the board room who make the tough calls on strategic choices."

Charles Prabakar, Strategy Leader, PepsiCo/Sears/Disney/Unisys

"The real thing! This book gave me the tools and insight to clearly understand and manage a very difficult situation. I appreciated reading the book. It helped a lot."

Roy Bateman, former member of three Boards of Directors.

"During my many years in leadership positions, I have seen first-hand the value of a collaborative approach with partners, clients, and stakeholders, along with a collaborative work environment. In fact, success increasingly co-incides with the ability to act in a collaborative fashion. Stephen Willis's new book is jam-packed with useful information and tools to succeed at making collaboration work. It is a real workhorse of a book - not the usual fluff and puff - and serves incredibly well with complex, tough situations."

David Anderson, Executive Director, San Francisco Zoo. Executive Director, Audubon Florida.

Stephen Willis takes a deep dive into the ways people work—or don't work—together. His concepts are as original as they are insightful. This book will help you size up your group members in terms of their inclination and motivation to collaborate."

Cindy Myers, Ph.D., CEO, Marin Services for Women

"Power through Collaboration is a thorough resource that provides a sound foundation and understanding of collaborative processes."

Marilyn Manning, Ph.D., CEO, The Consulting Team LLC. Author of 7 business books

Power through Collaboration

The Formula for Success in Challenging Situations!

Stephen Willis, Ph.D.

Power through Collaboration

The Formula for Success in Challenging Situations!

Books may be ordered through: www.willisllc.com

Willis Consulting LLC
4460-16 Redwood Hwy., #320
San Rafael, CA 94903
415-383-8555

V2.7 May 5, 2013

Customer service: this book is printed and distributed by Amazon and the Amazon subsidiary CreateSpace. Please contact Amazon or CreateSpace regarding any problems with printing quality or delivery.

ISBN: 0985476818
ISBN: 9780985476816

With loving appreciation I dedicate

this book to my daughter Kristina

Visit: www.willisllc.com

- Take the quick and easy online PtC Collaboration Scan that is discussed in this book, and receive a chart of your results. You can also arrange a consultation regarding your PtC Collaboration Scan results.

- Check out the comprehensive and advanced book *Power through Collaboration: When to Collaborate, Negotiate, or Dominate!* that this book is drawn from.

- Obtain information about the *Power through Collaboration* workshops:

  - Introduction to the 7-Step *Power through Collaboration* Model
  - Powering Up Team Performance via the *Collaboration Essentials*
  - Advanced *Power through Collaboration* for Complex and Difficult Situations
  - Stakeholder Analysis using the PtC Model

- Join our LinkedIn discussion group to benefit from helpful, useful, and engaging exchanges regarding collaboration.

- Sign up to receive the latest news about exciting *Power through Collaboration* developments; including our forthcoming series of eBooks and the *Power through Collaboration* app.

TABLE OF CONTENTS

PREFACE

Collaboration is much sought after, and for good reason. As our world becomes increasingly complex, interrelated, and connected, collaboration becomes ever more valuable and essential. Whenever you need the best results or face challenging and high-stakes situations, you need collaboration. Yet, collaboration is often poorly understood, and all too often ineffective.

Thus, the purpose of this book is to help you get to the heart of what collaboration is really all about. It sifts through the nuances, misconceptions, and confusions regarding collaboration. It examines common misconceptions that create problems, disappointments, and collaboration failures. It connects collaboration in its everyday role enabling everyday success, with its big picture potential as a mechanism for enabling larger scale social and economic success. It realistically confronts our dilemma of needing more collaboration but operating via self-interest.

It drills into the question of what aspects of collaboration are most reliably and truly determinative of collaboration success. The answer is definitely not cooperation as usual. The answer will likely be a new perspective for most people.

In our networked era of game-changing collaboration tools and technologies, the essence of collaboration is still about people. It is about how people feel about working together, and what makes them feel that way.

Another purpose of this book is to enable you to transform and operationalize the true essence of collaboration into the most effective and powerful form of human cooperation there is, that is, *Power through Collaboration.* Fortunately, there is a formula. The formula is built by taking a candid and realistic assessment of how different cooperation types, varying motivations, and the actual process of collaborating all interact to determine collaboration success versus failure. The PtC Formula alters choices, changes behavior, and enables successful collaboration.

This book is part of a series on *Power through Collaboration.* It is based on and drawn from my more comprehensive and advanced book *Power through Collaboration: When to Collaborate, Negotiate, or Dominate!* The advanced book can provide you with in-depth information about the *Power through Collaboration* Model, and how to use it to collaborate more successfully.

"Collaboration is essential,"
or so people echo.

"I am a great collaborator,"
or so people fantasize.

"Collaboration is all around us,"
or so people imagine.

"Collaboration is a core value in our company,"
or so people proclaim.

How many of these people really understand what collaboration is? Why do they experience so much confusion, angst, and disappointment when collaborating?

Common Misconceptions about Collaboration

Confusing Meanings and Nuances

Despite its value being highly touted and much talked about, collaboration often is unproductive or missing in action when needed the most. There are all too many examples of dramatic collaboration failures, both classic and current. I will name just a few. The Challenger space shuttle disaster. The Columbia space shuttle disaster. The 9/11 attack. The Iraq Weapons of Mass Destruction analysis. The response to Hurricane Katrina. The British Petroleum Deepwater Horizon explosion and oil spill. Collaboration failure was a contributing factor in all of these dramatic examples and led to disastrous consequences.

There are many reasons for such collaboration failures. One major reason is the pervasive lack of understanding regarding what collaboration truly is all about. Misconceptions regarding collaboration are a typical cause of collaboration problems and disappointment. Thus, this book examines the contradictions and confusion with respect to collaboration, and uncovers the real essence of collaboration.

The everyday meaning of collaboration appears to be different for different people. Whether considering one's own behavior or that of others, views of what collaboration entails often seem inconsistent and ambiguous.

Usually the differing views are at least "in the ballpark." Different terms are used to convey a meaning generally related to collaboration, such as "working together," "collaborative technologies," "teamwork," "cooperating together," "unity of purpose," "collective vision," "combined effort," "commitment to a group effort," "partnering," "collaborative relationships," "alliances," etcetera.

However, sometimes the differing meanings seem to be way out of the ballpark. Descriptions of collaborative behavior may not seem particularly collaborative – especially when people are describing their own supposedly collaborative behavior. The disparity between self-professed and actual behavior can have serious consequences. In critical situations a lack of real collaboration can put people on a collision course with disaster. Yet all the while those same people can mistakenly albeit sincerely hold themselves out as collaborating. People can be convinced that they are collaborating even though they have little understanding of what collaboration really entails. Most of us have seen and heard people insisting that their actions were collaborative when the evidence clearly suggested otherwise. Perhaps we have done so ourselves?

> With great sincerity, people can believe their actions are collaborative despite those with whom they are supposedly collaborating feeling exactly the opposite!

Naturally, the all too human capacity to be blind to our own behavior and its impacts is an obvious culprit behind the inconsistency and contradictions. Another chief suspect, often overlooked, is simply the confusion experienced about what collaboration actually is.

Collaborating can be complicated enough without parties having different understandings of what collaboration is all about. Effective collaboration does begin with and depend upon communication and understanding, starting especially with a shared understanding of the meaning of collaboration and what it entails. Achieving that shared understanding requires cutting through the confusion and sorting out common misconceptions about collaboration, and offering a clear definition of PtC collaboration. The Power through Collaboration (PtC) Model uses a specific meaning of collaboration that is very different from everyday usage.

When people experience confusion about what the term collaboration means, they are also reflecting confusion about what it does not mean. Peeling away the layers of confusion helps reveal the true core of collaboration. Taking a close look at what collaboration is not sharpens understanding of the essence of collaboration.

It also reveals common misconceptions that set the stage for collaboration difficulty and failure. So, as a prelude to unveiling the PtC definition of collaboration I will probe the common misconceptions and what collaboration is not.

1. Collaboration Is Not Just Cooperation

In the PtC Model collaboration is actually a subset of cooperation. It is one of three modes of cooperation. The other two are negotiation and domination, which are discussed further in my book "Power through Collaboration: When to Collaborate, Negotiate, or Dominate!"

People often do not distinguish between collaboration and cooperation. They seem to use the terms interchangeably in association with the act of working together; working on the same task or project; joint production of a product or service; the existence of common goals and mutual benefit; the process of how people work together; how well the people work together; people working together as equals; people feeling pressured to work together by necessity or coercion; and cost sharing and pooling of resources.

The act of working together seems to be the primary common component. It is often combined with the existence of common goals, and sometimes combined with the manner in which people work together. While working together and common goals indicate some degree of cooperation is occurring, it may not rise to the level of collaboration.

Despite the blurring of everyday usage, the PtC Model definition of collaboration is quite different from cooperation. Some differences show up even in everyday usage. For example, generic usage can refer to authors working together on a book as collaborating or as cooperating. Usage that is more specific narrows collaboration on a book to co-writing efforts, whereas cooperation opens up a wider range of actions which can involve anything from co-writing to typing to marketing. A person who cooperates in book delivery is not typically viewed as collaborating on the book.

Thus, collaboration is used to refer to a narrower range of cooperative behavior, and that behavior is considered to have a meaning related to partnering. I will have more to say about this throughout this book.

2. Collaboration Is Not Just the Act of Working Together

Working together is often proffered as a primary criterion for the occurrence of collaboration. It is far from sufficient. In and of itself the act of working together is not collaboration. People can readily work together without collaborating – something I see quite frequently. In fact, it is a major reason organizations request assistance! You probably see all around you non-collaborative working together.

People can be in the same room, even sitting right next to each other, and even working together on the same task or project, and still not be collaborating. They can just be interacting to whatever extent is demanded by the situation. Or they can just be putting on a show of appearing to cooperate without actually doing so. Picture people who bristle at the other's presence trying to collaborate. Or people who are compelled by economic necessity or brute force to work together. Although they may be working together, they are not likely to be collaborating, no matter how important the need!

Moreover, they are not likely to be highly productive. Merely working together in such situations usually does not lead to significant productivity or the desired results. Mistaking the mere act of working together on a task for collaboration can lead to the erroneous conclusion that collaboration is ineffective. The reality is the act of not collaborating is what is ineffective. Ironically, collaboration is often deemed ineffective when the real problem is a lack of collaboration.

3. Collaboration Does Not Mean Doing Everything Together

People can work alone or separately from each other, do separate tasks, have highly differentiated roles, be in different locations, or work via very different methods and processes, and still be collaborating. Some degree of working together typically occurs when collaborating, but it can vary considerably depending upon what is most effective for the task at hand.

Often working together on a task is not needed and is counterproductive. Working alone sometimes can be faster, cheaper, or produce the best results, and can still be part of collaborating.

4. Collaboration Is Not Just the Existence of Common Goals and Mutual Benefit

In numerous discussions I have had with people about what generates collaboration, common goals are mentioned most often as the basis for collaboration. In the PtC Model the mere existence of common goals and the prospect for mutual benefit are not necessarily an indicator that collaboration is occurring or will occur.

Common goals do present an opportunity and incentive for collaboration, and are often part of collaboration. Nevertheless, common goals alone are not a compelling promoter of collaboration.

Even the most obvious common goals and prospects for mutual benefit may not elicit collaboration. Financial, emotional, and physical battlefields are littered with trampled common goals. Bystanders and combatants alike are often frustrated that the wonderful common goals that they are clearly in sight get incessantly violated or completely ignored. People can have much to gain by working together, but may still work against, sabotage, and outright fight each other.

In the PtC Model, collaboration does not even require common goals and mutual benefit, despite common belief to the contrary. Collaboration can occur even when goals being worked on are not shared or of direct mutual benefit. I will address this further in subsequent chapters.

5. Collaboration Is Not Just Using Collaborative Tools and Processes, Teamwork, or Project Management

Innovative breakthroughs in collaboration technology are transforming how we connect, transact, work, and relate. Our understanding of and ability to utilize sophisticated communication and collaboration tools, well-designed teamwork templates, and advanced project management systems has never been greater.

Although highly valuable, such are not synonymous with collaboration. Just the fact of being technologically linked, connected, or networked is not equivalent to nor a substitute for collaboration. No matter how advanced or sophisticated, collaboration tools and processes themselves cannot produce collaboration. Without a doubt they play an invaluable supportive role, but collaboration is first and foremost about people.

A manager at a Fortune 100 company well known for its use of collaboration tools and processes described it to me this way:

> "… most of us on the team are 'remote' …. My projects have included working with colleagues and partners in India, Japan, China as well as many locations across the US. Sometimes computer based collaboration -- synchronous (IM) and asynchronous (email and social environments) -- must be augmented with voice (phone) and sometimes with the ability to point to something in common and say, 'See, that is what I'm talking about...' or watch the expression on someone's face as they talk about an issue or a challenge (video conferencing). The real issue comes down to how motivated are the participants to SHARE information with each other -- to want to give as much as they get from each other. That is the key to it. Sometimes the tools help -- sometimes they can interfere."

Even the best collaboration tools and processes can be ignored, thwarted, or misused. If so motivated, people who are indifferent or opposed to the goals of a team or organization can endure or utilize seemingly collaborative processes, but without producing significant results. People can put on a good show and just go through the motions. Even people in outright conflict can strategically engage in seemingly collaborative processes, but actually be working against each other or trying to gain an unfair advantage. In such situations, the collaboration tools and processes are often blamed for the collaboration failure. Or the very concept of collaboration is viewed as flawed and unworkable. In reality, the supposed collaboration was only a façade and never actually existed.

> Lion prides often display excellent teamwork when hunting, but despite their triumphant team prowess, such predators are not collaborating.

Most organizational activities can be accomplished without genuine collaboration, such as: establishing mission, goals, roles, responsibilities, and accountability; communicating and sharing knowledge and information; establishing timelines and critical paths; developing success strategies and action plans; building consensus on critical issues; decision making and problem solving; engaging stakeholders; obtaining and allocating resources; aligning strategy and operations; etcetera.

Such organizational processes are all components of effective cooperation. They are necessary for the success of most ventures, and are typically undertaken with a collaborative appearance. Thus, they are commonly equated with collaboration, and have become de facto indicators of collaboration in operation. Yet, these processes and proscribed behaviors of collaboration can all be done without real collaboration. Just about every collaborative appearing behavior and process can readily be part of non-collaboration, and sometimes even part of predation.

Our revolutionary collaboration technology and processes are not inherently collaborative. They are merely tools at our disposal with the potential to facilitate and serve genuine collaborative purposes, or exactly the opposite. They can be used to achieve dramatically non-collaborative results, including attempting to control and dominate, to more effectively do battle, or to more effectively wreak destruction.

> Collaboration 2.0 has the potential to expand collaboration, but also enables modern day breakthroughs in the power to exploit, prey on, and enslave people.

6. Collaboration Is Not Collaborationism

Cooperation with the Nazis during World War II was referred to as collaboration, and thus associated the term collaboration with betrayal and cooperating with an enemy. The type of cooperation produced by the threats, oppression, and brutal coercion of the Nazis is not at all related to PtC Model collaboration.

Today a sizable majority of the population has no negative connotation of the term collaboration. On the Internet collaboration is an exciting buzzword for working together that is powered by innovative tools and technology. Although dictionaries reference the negative connotation, many people are barely familiar with the past pejorative usage. They may even encounter the World War II usage in movies or books, but not notice a contradiction with present day usage.

To bridge the reality of a previous era with a current era, 'collaborationism' and 'collaborationist' are used for the cooperative behavior displayed with or coerced by the Nazis, thereby freeing up 'collaboration' and 'collaborator' for its contemporary positive meaning.

7. Collaboration Does Not Mean the Absence of Differences, Disagreements, or Conflict

Collaboration often fosters greater cohesion and harmony, but that does not mean having to be polite, nice, and agreeable to everyone all the time. The absence of conflict is neither required for nor indicative of collaboration, and can sometimes indicate the opposite.

> Collaboration is about getting results, not kumbaya.

A harmonious facade can imply that disagreements or conflicting interests feel too daunting to face, and are being avoided. Strained politeness may reflect fear of looking below the surface, or a concern about conflict getting out of control. Alternatively, polite and agreeable behavior can actually be a deception. A common predator tactic is to carefully restrain emotions and behavior so as not to spook the quarry and precipitate outright "fight or flight" which would jeopardize an advantageous position.

A facade of harmony that prevents crucial issues from being addressed can be detrimental. As Edwin Land, the co-founder of the Polaroid Corporation, stated, "Politeness is the poison of collaboration." Yet politeness is a common substitute when genuine collaboration is lacking or difficult to obtain.

Another common substitute for collaboration is focusing on *alignment* as a means of reducing conflict and disagreement around goals. Despite being an inadequate substitute, it is often rolled out as collaboration. It is not. Alignment can be purchased with monetary incentives, cajoled by group pressure, or imposed through coercion. Such pseudo-alignment squelches important voices, ideas, and options. It can produce groupthink, diminished adaptability, stymied innovation, and seriously flawed decisions. Alignment without real collaboration can be disastrous.

Collaboration does not involve getting everyone to look, think, and behave alike. Collaboration does involve people contributing their different thinking and behaviors to the effort of achieving each other's goals, which are sometimes shared in common, and sometimes not. Collaboration allows many voices and ideas, and works with them.

Collaboration takes diverse viewpoints and progresses from tolerating them to understanding, respecting, balancing, integrating, and ultimately synthesizing them. Differences and diversity become an opportunity to move ahead and explore new territory, rather than to hold on or retreat to the familiar. Indeed effective collaboration approaches conflict as a potential source of new ideas, new options, and off the radar opportunities.

> Regardless of whether or not conflict is useful or necessary, it is inevitable. Collaboration is not a state of perfection and does not change the inevitability of conflict.

A manageable degree of tension, conflict, and competition can be productive for the workings of organizations. However, the positive or negative value of conflict as compared to harmony is not the same for every situation. Rather, it is determined by the nature of the goals to be accomplished, the extent to which viewpoints converge or clash, and what is at stake. For example, if the stakes are low, then conflict can be sidestepped. If the stakes are high, avoiding conflict can be costly. All too often, people operate according to the reverse notion. When it is imperative to achieve the best possible outcome, conflict needs to be faced and managed productively.

The best approach, for collaborative situations is to make conflict purposeful and productive, and harness its potential for creating innovative options and solutions. In general, collaboration allows for better use and management of conflict. It creates a safer climate in which to deal directly with sensitive and divisive issues. Collaborators tend to have greater toleration for differences of opinion, greater ability working around or resolving people related conflicts, and staying focused on what really needs to be accomplished.

8. Collaboration Does Not Require Being Leaderless and Egalitarian

Organizational structure is important for but not determinative of the degree of collaboration. Collaboration can occur in very different organizational structures.

Collaboration is not synonymous with an absence or diminishment of leaders, or the elimination of hierarchy. Although collaboration is often associated with flatter organizations, less rigid hierarchies, egalitarian norms, consensus decision making, and decentralized power and authority, such is not always the case. None of these is an essential defining component of collaboration.

Even the most egalitarian structure is no guarantee that collaboration will occur. Egalitarian organizations can be overwhelmed by conflict and completely devoid of collaboration.

> Collaboration is more important for the success of a given organizational structure than a given structure is for the success of collaboration.

Organizational structure and processes can promote and guide collaboration, but cannot assure it. Collaboration opens the door to the numerous foibles of human personality, interactions, and relationships. Such are not abolished by even the most idealistic organizational structure and process. Organizational structure can discourage troublesome behaviors and promote effective cooperation only to the extent that people's personality types and motivations allow. The particular types and motivations involved trump and readily over-ride structure and process. Collaborative potential must exist at the level of type and motivation in order to be actualized via organizational structure and process.

With a favorable mix of personality types and motivations, collaboration can occur within organizational structures that range from highly equalitarian to highly hierarchical, including the military, and can occur between and across the highest to the lowest levels. Collaboration allows for decision making to be conducted via consensus or via authorized and centralized leaders or a chain of command. Even collaborative organizations can require centralized leadership to succeed. Success is determined more by extent of collaboration than by type of leadership structure.

> When authoritative or centralized leadership is needed, collaboration is a vital part of the process of enabling such leadership and making it effective.

Leadership is usually exerted very differently in collaborative compared to autocratic organizations. Taskmasters and micro-managers are not needed because people in collaborative organizations are more likely to be motivated enough to take the initiative and do what needs to be done.

Without highly visible reliance on domination or prodding of stereotypical leaders, collaborative organizations can appear leaderless from the outside. Flexible or informal leadership roles that morph and shift from person to person as tasks require are easy to miss. Leaders can be effective and essential, but less visible to those who do not understand how things get done in collaborative organizations.

In collaborative yet hierarchical organizations, leaders may be more obvious, but still function differently from non-collaborative counterparts. When collaboratively functioning leaders make decisions, those affected typically feel understood, respected, and appropriately involved. They experience goodwill and trust with respect to the designated leader's decision-making efforts and intentions.

9. Collaboration Does Not Involve Being Weak, Ineffective, or Powerless

Collaboration is often viewed as lacking significant power. The act of collaboration is often construed as a sign of weakness. It is deemed something to do when you do not have or do not need real power.

Power is historically associated with the capability to have control over other people and make them do what you want them to do. Thus, power is equated with some form of domination, and negotiation is viewed as an adjunct to domination.

Equating power with domination is a natural outgrowth of domination's successful track record at compelling cooperation. Humans dominating humans has been a consistently rewarding practice throughout evolution. Democratic or participatory governance has been relatively infrequent by comparison. Our contemporary universal suffrage is rare, incessantly resisted, and deviously undermined. Domination is more prevalent in our national and local governance than collaboration.

The power of domination cannot be overstated. For eons entire civilizations have been successfully created and routinely operated via domination and coercion. Just about every major country established an empire at one time or another.

To emphasize the point I will name just a few: the Roman Empire, the Macedonian Empire, the Byzantine Empire, the Persian Empire, the Egyptian Dynasties, the Neo-Assyrian Empire, the Ottoman Empire, the Umayyad Caliphate, the Abbasid Caliphate, the Rashidun Caliphate, the Mongol Empire, the Napoleonic empire, the British Empire, the Russian Empire, the Spanish Empire, the French Empire, the Portuguese Empire, the Japanese Empire, the Tibetan Empire, the Qing Dynasty, the Yuan Dynasty, the Ming Dynasty, the Han Dynasty, the Inca Empire, the Aztec Empire, etcetera. The reigns of kings, queens, emperors, rajahs, maharajahs, czars, and sultans all operated via domination. For centuries various forms of slavery and servitude were a highly successful means of building wealth and power for the Romans, Mongols, Egyptians, Spaniards, Americans, British, etc.

Despite historical reliance on domination as the primary mode of exerting power, it is counterproductive and an obstacle to success in a highly developed and advanced society. In the more complex context of contemporary times, real power is the power to act with other people. That is what collaboration is all about.

> The ability to collaborate and work with others toward a goal is more powerful and can accomplish so much more than the ability to control and make people do what you want them to do.

Working with people can achieve so much more than trying to make them do what needs to be done. Collaboration gets results. Ironically, power over and against other people can be counterproductive by actually reducing the power to accomplish what needs to be accomplished.

Collaboration is the exact opposite of weakness and powerlessness. Collaboration is the most powerful means of getting things done and achieving important goals.

10. Collaboration Does Not Require Giving Up Self-Identity and Personal Power

A common misconception is to equate gaining power through collaboration with a corresponding bee-like or ant-like loss of individual self-identity and self-power.

Some people point to social species such as bees and ants as models on which to base human collaboration. The reliable, acquiescent, and orderly cooperation of bees and ants can seem appealing. The seeming simplicity and dedication of worker bees and ant drones contrast starkly with the nuances and fickleness of human cooperation. Many companies and countries attempt to obtain cooperation via downgrading human potential to the limited potential of bees and ants. Should they succeed, they often regret it, and spend a lot of resources trying to undo it.

When I hear people suggest human cooperation should be based on automatic and reflexive behavior like that of bees and ants, they sound well-intentioned. Yet, they seem unaware of the disconcerting implications. Advocating that humans should cooperate like bees or ants implies a preference for people being docile, obedient, and doing exactly what they are instinctively programmed to do.

Cooperative behavior that abandons human consciousness and capability is not a competitive advantage, especially for companies and countries that need to survive in complex circumstances, or need to create, innovate, progress, and evolve. Given the complexity and challenges involved in contemporary business survival, would you rather have your fate rest in the hands of people functioning as worker bees and ant drones, or as fully empowered and motivated human beings?

True, bees and ants have been successful and thriving species for at least as long as humans have. They are clearly superb at what they do. Ironically, they may even outlast humans! No slight toward bees and ants is intended, but despite their orderly and reliable cooperation, the degree of evolutionary advancement of bees and ants is relatively stagnant.

Their level of accomplishment and their capability to deal with complexity are far below that of humans. They are well adapted to the niches that they function in, but they are not at the top of the earth food chain as humans are. They do not visit the moon and probe outer space; explore the depths of the oceans; transverse continents by plane; perform heart and kidney transplants; or create art, science, and literature. In addition, the ant and bee understanding of complex business models, strategies, and operations is far below that of humans.

Humans perform and achieve at a much higher level than bees and ants. Too much is lost if humans function as bees and ants. If humans do so, however cooperatively, they are incurring a dramatic capability downgrade that is a prescription for mediocrity and failure.

The instinct driven cooperative behavior of bees and ants is not considered collaboration in the PtC Model. Some think that it is. They view collaboration as each individual subordinating their individual power and identify to group and collective dictates. They view collaboration as antagonistic to individual empowerment – as group power trumping individual power. They argue either for or against the need to sacrifice individual identity on the altar of collaboration for the collective good.

Actually, the opposite is the case. Engagement and social adaptation via the process of collaboration involves empowered individuals working willingly and freely toward mutually identified goals, sometimes together as a group and sometimes separately as individuals.

> Power through Collaboration is completely dependent upon individual empowerment for its success.

Any form of social engagement requires some degree of compromise, but collaboration does not require nor benefit from burdensome compromising and capitulation. Collaboration is not synonymous with giving up power and being weak and defenseless. It is not just being agreeable or obsequious. It is not about always accommodating, conceding, *rolling over*, and *giving in and going along*. It is not about obedience to the preferences or dictates of a group or larger community. Indeed such behavior is more typical of enslavement or of cooperative behavior coerced by force or economic necessity.

Disempowered individuals are not capable of working *willingly and freely*. Consequently, they are much less effective as potential collaborators. Collaboration withers away whenever people are not empowered.

In fact, successful collaboration requires and benefits from the assertive contributions of fully empowered people to generate the best results. Collaboration thrives on and needs empowered individuals who are capable of working *willingly and freely*. Individual empowerment enhances collaboration. The more you have of the former, the more you have of the latter as well.

In contrast to routine, coerced, or instinct-driven cooperation, genuine collaboration not only requires, but also creates and supports individual empowerment. An intrinsic hallmark and reliable indicator of real collaboration is the fact that it is empowering! Collaboration nurtures and brings out strong personal power, which in turn, nurtures collaboration.

We live in an increasingly complex world where individuals relying solely on their own innate abilities and talents cannot achieve anything of significance. Even those fortunate enough to be born with a foundation of great potential. Potential remains untapped potential unless developed. All of us depend on the nurturing, support, and influence of the surrounding social system for the development of our personal capabilities.

> It is a lack of collaboration in a society that causes a diminished self-identity and a loss of personal power.

Our self-identity and personal power originate and grow within our social system. Long gone are the days when a person could develop aside from the dominant and advanced social system, and end up with significant personal power within or aside from it. The requirements for success are now too complicated. There is too much complex material to master and learn from others. Learning at an advanced level from the surrounding network of people and the social system is required.

A strong self-identity and personal power are created and enhanced via a collaborative culture. Collaboration not only optimizes the capability of groups, organizations, and societies, but also of individuals. It encourages and enables people to use their capabilities to their maximum potential. Without collaboration, individuals cannot accomplish all that they are capable of accomplishing via collaboration.

Phil Jackson was named one of the ten greatest coaches in the history of the National Basketball Association (NBA), and inducted into the Basketball Hall of Fame. He has the highest winning percentage of any NBA coach, and holds the NBA record for winning the most championships. He is also the author of several team and strategy books. This championship player and coach concludes:[1]

> "The strength of the team is each individual member. The strength of each member is the team."

Without collaboration, individuals cannot accomplish all that they are capable of accomplishing via collaboration. For example, a top producing sales executive was continuously surpassing his own sales records. The executive took great pride in his personal success even though the sales department that he headed was doing poorly, and his company was losing money. While exploring the reasons his company was in trouble, the executive complained about his salespeople competing with and working against him. He tellingly smugly bragged about outsmarting them and doing better than them in spite of their attempts to sabotage his success.

The executive used a dominating approach in his futile attempts to boost productivity from his sales force. He felt it was him versus them, and that they needed to operate his way. He resisted collaborating with them, feeling that to do so would weigh him down and undermine his own success. He could not envision that they could all work together collaboratively to be top producers, much less that other sales team members could actually help him be even more successful.

The concept of an empowered team of All-Stars in which each team member enables the others to perform at their personal best was foreign to him. Yet, it was just what he needed for his company to be successful again. Eventually, it was a collaboratively functioning team of All-Stars that enabled both he and the company to be more financially successful than they ever had been.

> The more difficult, complex, and vital the task is, the more essential as well as advantageous collaboration of empowered individuals actually is.

Especially when highly effective performance and outstanding results are called for, mere cooperation is usually not enough. Collaboration of empowered people is the most powerful, and sometimes the only way, to succeed.

11. Collaboration Is Not Forced Cooperation

There is a clear distinction between cooperation and collaboration with respect to the use of and reliance on coercion. Cooperation can be obtained via coercion and domination. Someone being arrested may cooperate with police commands for fear of being forcefully subdued. A child may obey a parent's *request* to go to bed to avoid implied punishment. An employee may *volunteer* for unpaid overtime for fear of being fired. Cooperation elicited by police, parents, or employers by virtue of their controlling or dominating position and power, is not viewed as collaboration. "You better cooperate or else" is not considered a prelude to collaboration, only cooperation. Coercion is not conducive to and readily stifles collaboration.

Coercion, whether by economic necessity or by brute force, cannot turn working together on the same task into collaboration. Coerced people are unlikely to collaborate to achieve the designated goals no matter how interrelated their tasks. When coercion is used to compel collaboration, the only collaborative aspect to working together may be covert efforts to sabotage the work at hand.

Similarly, coercion by economic necessity or brute force, cannot convert having similar individual goals or common goals into collaboration. Even if coercion creates common goals, genuine collaboration will be elusive or an expedient facade. Common goals created by coercion can get people to work together, but unwillingly. Common goals may motivate working together, but not collaboration.

Similarly, coercion cannot make people with clashing personalities, irritating work habits, or conflicting values collaborate. Coercion can make them work together to achieve the same goal just because they think they can obtain more of what they want than by working alone. Or they want to avoid an unwanted or punitive consequence. Such pressured situations are not conducive to collaboration.

> Whereas cooperation can be either coerced or voluntary, collaboration can only be voluntary.

Resorting to coercion or domination implies the absence of collaboration. When people negotiate or make accommodations with dominating or controlling parties it is not collaboration, just a form of cooperation.

This distinction can be seen in the cooperation of social predators such as lions that manifest intensive levels of cooperative teamwork when hunting. But, lion prides do not collaborate. They are manifesting effective cooperation that is predominantly survival driven, and implemented by means of domination and power.

The post-hunting behavior of the lion pride is a telling indicator of just how collaborative they really are. The pride does not share the kill according to need or merit. Feasting on the spoils of the hunt is an *everyone for themself* affair. How much, and whether or not any particular animal gets to eat at all, is determined solely by what that animal can command for themself. The less powerful only get to eat after the more powerful and dominant have satisfied themselves. If there is not enough of the kill to go around, then those who cannot command a portion for themselves, no matter how young, old, or in need, do not get to eat – and die.

12. Collaboration Is Not Just Intensive Cooperation

Intensive cooperation does not automatically become collaboration. Often extensive and intertwined forms of cooperation, such as strategic alliances and joint ventures, are referred to as *collaborations*. However, both cooperation and collaboration can involve either a minimal or an extensive relationship. The extent of common goals and mutual benefit can vary from a little to a lot. The degree of involvement can range from informal working together; to simple verbal agreements; to limited service agreements; to coordinated service delivery; to joint product development; to strategic alliances; or to joint ventures. The arrangement can be either informal or made tightly binding and strictly enforced.

Both cooperating or collaborating organizations and individuals may maintain complete autonomy, or build an integrated organizational structure and system with shared power and authority. Both allow for minimal to nearly complete integration with respect to roles and authority, planning and implementation, scope of mission and goals, policy and procedures, decision-making and communication processes, pooling resources, assuming risks, etcetera.

Just because cooperation is extensive and intensive does not make it collaboration. The mistake of erroneously assuming a joint venture is a collaboration is a typical source of serious problems. Many a joint venture is in reality at best a cooperation based on negotiation or domination, and sometimes not even that. Mere cooperative behavior is often given the halo of collaboration.

> The more extensive and integrated the cooperative endeavor, the more vital it is that it be collaborative. And the more risk if it is not.

Collaboration is the ultimate source of power.

Whereas cooperation functions like standard octane fuel for driving work performance, collaboration functions like rocket fuel for propelling performance to stratospheric heights. Collaboration is the super-charged fuel for outstanding accomplishments.

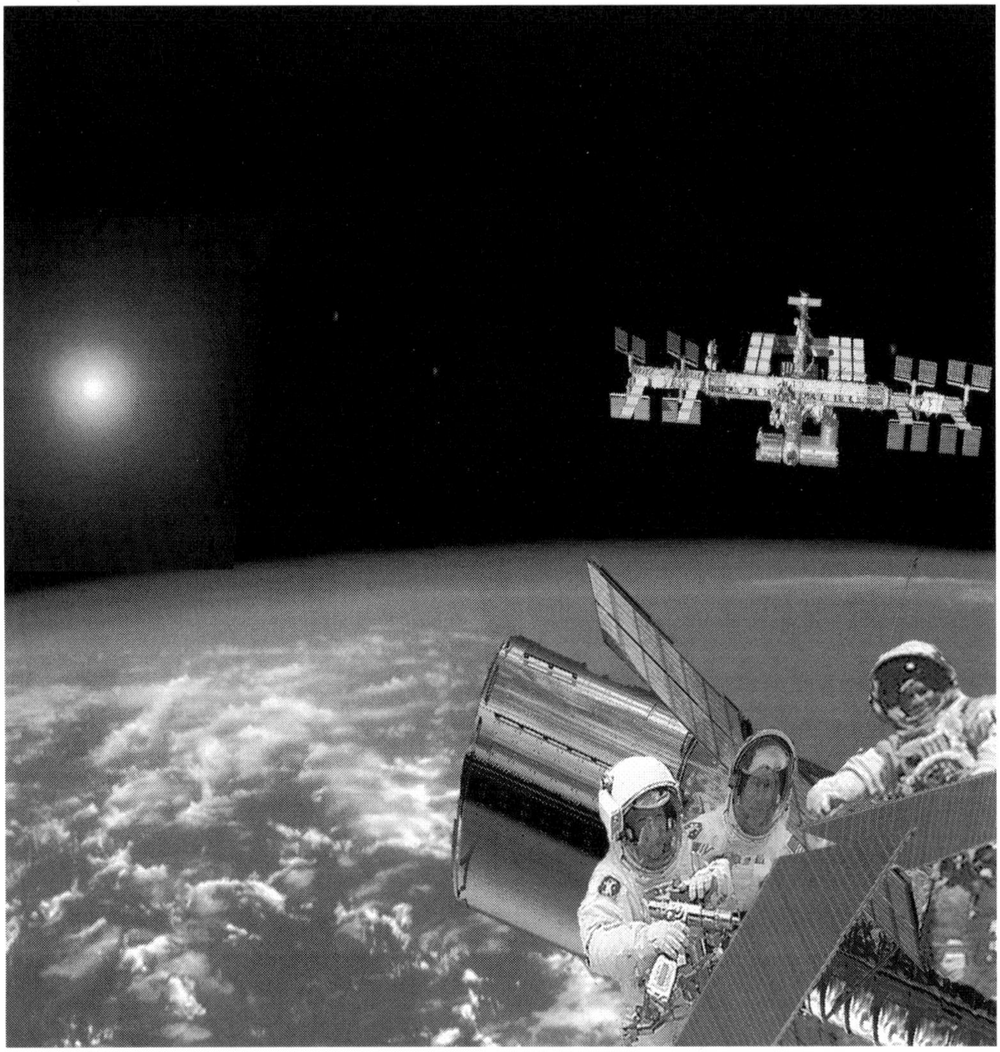

The Real Essence of Collaboration

Collaboration Is Much More Powerful Then Cooperation

In my experience, as cooperation becomes more intensive, gains in performance effectiveness and goal attainment increase, until reaching a point of diminishing returns, and then decrease. A high level of cooperation is better than none or just a little, but its relative effectiveness decreases. In contrast, collaboration produces steadily increasing performance effectiveness and goal attainment with no drop-off, as illustrated in the following **Effectiveness & Goal Attainment: Collaboration vs Cooperation** diagram.

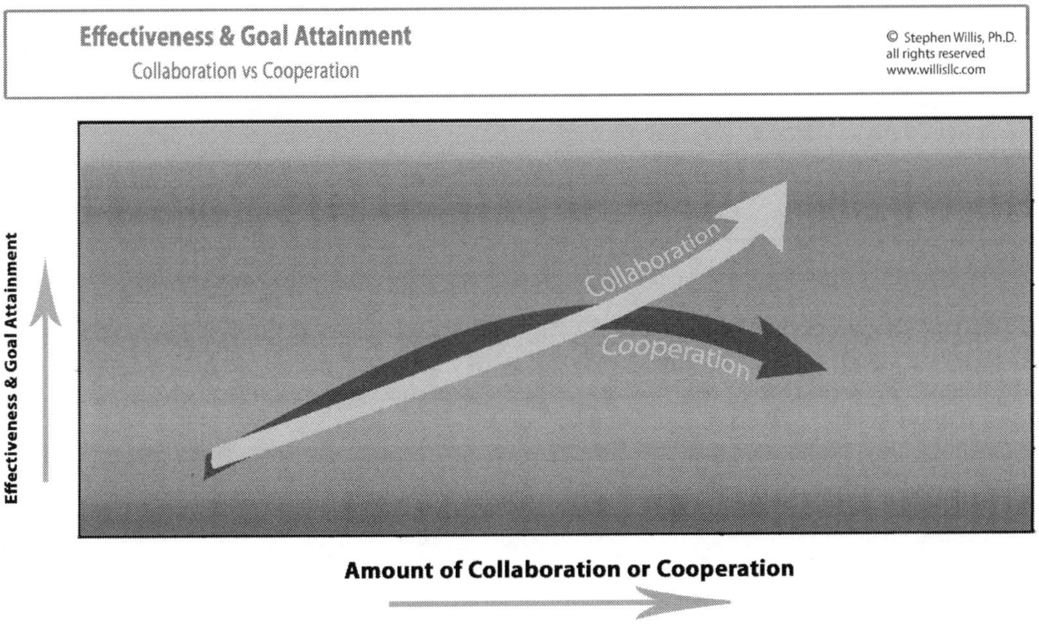

The drop-off in gains from cooperation is due to common people issues. Ordinary cooperation is often plagued by friction around: differing ideas, strategies, and tactics; power, control, and competition; status, prestige, rank, or worth; who deserves and is paid more; and so on. Cooperating parties often have: competing interests and goals; people focused only on their own goals; people using pretexts and conflicts to gain an advantage; and difficulty tolerating diversity regarding gender, sexual orientation, ethnic, racial, religious, and philosophical differences.

With routine cooperation, such stresses more readily lead to conflict, which more readily leads to combat, which more readily leads to not facing difficult issues than is the case for collaboration. Excessive conflict avoidance and overly agreeable or obsequious behavior degrade performance and results. So does a complete lack of conflict avoidance that leads to poorly managed and excessive conflict.

Additionally, the process and results of ordinary cooperation are less productive than for collaboration. Decisions, solutions, and actions can fall short of expectations, and create disappointment. In hindsight, the gap between what could have been and the actual results feeds regret and frustration.

Collaboration is not immune to such common frictions and disappointments, but does provide a protective effect because of the support for individual empowerment that is integral to collaborating; the mechanism by which people with collaborative dispositions operate; and the motivations that drive them. Thus, collaboration frees people from the constraints of routine cooperation. Collaboration allows, motivates, and enables people to work together at their best.

Thus, the more cooperation you have or need, the messier it can become. The more collaboration you have or need, the better it can become.

Not every enterprise can be, nor need be collaborative. Collaboration is not something to do all the time. It is just one of many organizational characteristics determined by mission, type of people involved and their motivations, and the particular circumstances. Everyday cooperation is valuable and useful. It can be cost effective with respect to time and money, can achieve many constructive purposes, and is often sufficient for everyday tasks. However, it sometimes is not up to the demands of the job, and falls far short of *Power through Collaboration*.

When collaboration is deployed, it is the most powerful mechanism for overcoming challenges, dealing with complexity, driving innovation, and achieving vital goals. The typical cooperation most people operate by and settle for cannot compare to collaboration. Collaboration creates and accomplishes to an extent that mere cooperation can never hope for or dream of.

Whenever the best results are needed -- collaboration is needed:

- Decisive strategies
- Successful decisions
- Top performing teams
- Workable reorganizations
- Effective change initiatives
- Innovative ideas and products
- Efficient supply chain processes
- Viable solutions and agreements
- Value-added mergers & acquisitions
- Productive stakeholder engagements
- Rewarding alliances and joint ventures
- Accomplishing critically important missions

Collaboration is the ultimate source of power. Whereas cooperation functions like standard octane fuel for driving work performance, collaboration functions like rocket fuel for propelling work performance to stratospheric heights. It is the supercharged fuel for great accomplishments. That is why this book is entitled *Power through Collaboration.*

By now you might be thinking, "What is this collaboration that is so powerful, and where do I get some?" So, let us now focus on what collaboration is.

Collaboration is a subset of goal directed cooperative behavior in which people mutually care about achieving each other's goals and work willingly and freely to achieve each other's goals.

The Key Components of Collaboration

Considering that the generic *working toward a goal* is a given, the key components of the above definition of collaboration are:

- mutually care about achieving each other's goals
- work to achieve each other's goals
- willingly and freely

All three components are required for cooperative behavior to be deemed collaboration in the PtC Model. Working *willingly and freely* is usually viewed as a core component of collaboration. The use of coercion rules out collaboration. Coercion can compel cooperation, but not working willingly and freely to achieve each other's goals. Slave laborers can be forced to cooperate, but not to collaborate. They neither work willingly and freely, nor care about achieving a dominator's goals, and often care about *not* achieving them.

As long as people do not feel coerced, even rigidly hierarchical organizations with highly defined authority structures, such as the military, can function collaboratively. Lower as well as higher ranked personnel can care about and work willingly and freely to achieve the organization's mission and goals.

Working willingly and freely to achieve each other's goals goes hand-in-hand with mutual caring about achieving each other's goals. The latter is an essential component. Without it there can be no collaboration. There can be cooperation, but not collaboration.

Collaboration is goal directed work, but common goals are not necessary for collaboration to occur. Common goals are typical, yet nonessential. Goals of collaborators can be completely shared, somewhat overlapping, or separate and distinct. Regardless of the extent to which goals overlap, collaboration is caring about and working to achieve the goals of all significant collaborators and stakeholders, not just one's own goals or goals shared in common.

Following is a quick and easy to take PtC Collaboration Scan based on the three components of the PtC collaboration definition. It can help you assess and more directly discuss the level of PtC collaboration by which you operate.

PtC Collaboration Scan (beta):

Think of a person, group, or organization that you are collaborating with, or might collaborate with. Write a nickname for them in the blank spaces below. For each question, select one answer that seems most accurate to you. Then circle the number to the right of that answer. You will add up the numbers when you are finished. If you are not yet collaborating, then answer according to what you expect if you were to collaborate with them.

1. When working with ________________________, how much do you care about achieving their goals?

I want <u>very much</u> to achieve their goals.	....	3
I want <u>somewhat</u> to achieve their goals.	....	2
I want <u>slightly</u> to achieve their goals.	....	1
I am neutral about achieving their goals.	....	0
I want <u>slightly</u> *not* to achieve their goals.	....	-1
I want <u>somewhat</u> *not* to achieve their goals.	....	-2
I want <u>very much</u> *not* to achieve their goals.	....	-3

2. When working with ________________________, how much do you work to achieve their goals?

I work <u>very much</u> to achieve their goals.	....	3
I work <u>somewhat</u> to achieve their goals.	....	2
I work <u>slightly</u> to achieve their goals.	....	1
I work neither for nor against achieving their goals.	....	0
I work <u>slightly</u> *against* achieving their goals.	....	-1
I work <u>somewhat</u> *against* achieving their goals.	....	-2
I work <u>very much</u> *against* achieving their goals.	....	-3

3. When or if you were to work to achieve ________________________ goals, do you do so willingly and freely?

<u>Very</u> willingly and freely.	....	3
<u>Somewhat</u> willingly and freely.	....	2
<u>Slightly</u> willingly and freely.	....	1
Neither willingly/freely nor *un*willingly/*non*-freely.	....	0
<u>Slightly</u> *un*willingly and *non*-freely.	....	-1
<u>Somewhat</u> *un*willingly and *non*-freely.	....	-2
<u>Very much</u> *un*willingly and *non*-freely.	....	-3

4. When working with ________________________, how much do they care about achieving your goals?

They want very much to achieve my goals.	....	3
They want somewhat to achieve my goals.	....	2
They want slightly to achieve my goals.	....	1
They are neutral about achieving my goals.	....	0
They want slightly *not* to achieve my goals.	....	-1
They want somewhat *not* to achieve my goals.	....	-2
They want very much *not* to achieve my goals.	....	-3

5. When working with _________________________, how much do they work to achieve your goals?

They work very much to achieve my goals.	....	3
They work somewhat to achieve my goals.	....	2
They work slightly to achieve my goals.	....	1
They work neither for nor against achieving my goals.	....	0
They work slightly *against* achieving my goals.	....	-1
They work somewhat *against* achieving my goals.	....	-2
They work very much *against* achieving my goals.	....	-3

6. When or if __________________________ were to work to achieve your goals, do they do so willingly and freely?

Very willingly and freely.	....	3
Somewhat willingly and freely.	....	2
Slightly willingly and freely.	....	1
Neither willingly/freely nor *un*willingly/*non*-freely.	....	0
Slightly *un*willingly and *non*-freely.	....	-1
Somewhat *un*willingly and *non*-freely.	....	-2
Very much *un*willingly and *non*-freely.	....	-3

Just add your 6 scores to obtain your **PtC Collaboration Scan Total:** _______

Total scores can range from -18 (least collaborative) to 0 (neutral) to +18 (most collaborative).

- Also, you can compare your responses on each of the individual questions.
- Also, you can have others you are working with take the scan and compare their total score as well as responses on individual questions with yours.

Example of Alex and Chris. To illustrate comparing the PtC Collaboration Scan responses of two collaborating parties, I will use the example of Alex and Chris. Although they had a need to work closely with each other, they were having serious difficulties collaborating.

Their scan profile provided clues regarding what Alex and Chris needed to discuss and work on to improve their collaboration effectiveness. Their scan profile is illustrated in the following **Collaboration Scan: Alex and Chris** diagram.

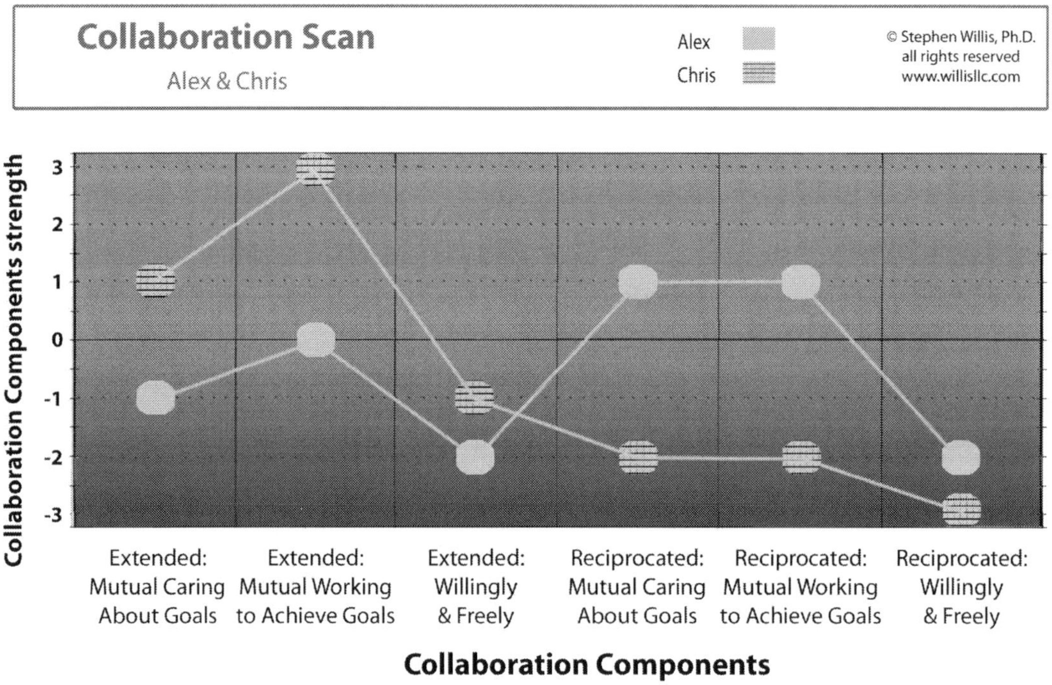

The Collaboration Scan diagram shows that most of Alex and Chris's scores are in negative territory below the 0 line. Specifically:

Mutual caring about achieving each other's goals. The extent of *mutual caring about each other's goals* that is *Extended* by Alex and Chris toward each other is problematic. Alex does not care about achieving Chris's goals, and in fact, *slightly* wants not to achieve Chris's goals. Chris only *slightly* cares about achieving Alex's goals.

In addition, the extent of *mutual caring about each other's goals* that is perceived as *Reciprocated* by Alex and Chris from each other is problematic. Alex perceives that Chris only *slightly* cares about achieving Alex's goals. And Chris perceives that Alex *somewhat* wants not to achieve Chris's goals.

Mutual working to achieve each other's goals. The extent of *mutual working to achieve each other's goals* that is *Extended* by Alex and Chris toward each other is out of balance and also problematic. Alex does not work to achieve Chris's goals. Yet, Chris reports working very *much* to achieve Alex's goals.

The *mutual working to achieve each other's goals* that is perceived as *Reciprocated* by Alex and Chris from each other is also problematic. Alex perceives that Chris only *slightly* works to achieve Alex's goals, which contradicts Chris's feeling of working *very much* to achieve Alex's goals. The discrepancy leads to Chris's feeling that working hard to benefit Alex is unappreciated and a wasted effort. Chris's perception that Alex works against achieving Chris's goals also undermines Chris's motivation to collaborate.

Working willingly and freely to achieve each other's goals. With regard to *Extended*, the extent to which Alex and Chris work willingly and freely is also problematic. If or when they might work to achieve each other's goals, neither does so willingly and freely. Alex does not work at all to achieve Chris's goals, and if Alex were to, it would be *somewhat* unwillingly and non-freely. Chris does work to achieve Alex's goals, but does so *slightly* unwillingly and non-freely.

Regarding *Reciprocated*, both perceive that any working to achieve each other's goals is only done unwillingly and non-freely. Alex perceives that Chris's working to achieve Alex's goals is done *somewhat* unwillingly and non-freely. Chris perceives that if Alex were to work to achieve Chris's goals, that it would be *very much* unwillingly and non-freely.

Collaboration Scan Totals:

- Alex: -3.0
- Chris: -4.0
- Average: -3.5

Averaging Alex and Chris's total scores produces a PtC Collaboration Scan Total of -3.5. This places them in negative territory within the range of 18 to -18, with 0 being neutral. Effective PtC Collaboration with such a scan profile is challenging.

The PtC Collaboration Scan is also available online. Just go to the survey page at the following website and follow the instructions:

www.willisllc.com/survey

- You can take the PtC Collaboration Scan online.
- You can have an entire group take the scan and have your responses grouped together.
- You can select the option to receive a diagram of your results.
- You can receive a telephone consultation regarding the meaning of the scan results, and explore what options and actions are indicated for your situation.

A Pivotal Shift

The centrality of mutual caring about achieving each other's goals instead of achieving common goals is for some a perplexing shift. It has significant implications that will be evident throughout this book. Those looking for another pat recipe of well-defined and proscribed collaborative behaviors to better achieve common goals may end up being disappointed.

The latter's quest is futile because without the essential foundation of mutual caring about achieving each other's goals, the plethora of recipes for collaboration produce sour results. Every potential common goal can be ignored or abandoned due to changing circumstances. All too often I have seen the most promising and mutually beneficial common goals languish from neglect. The parties cannot agree to work on the common goals for their mutual benefit. Or their efforts are halfhearted and ineffective. Or the goals remain separate goals of separate parties. The parties merely have the same individual goals, but do not share them in common. Additionally, without mutual caring about each other's goals just about every collaborative appearing behavior can readily be part of non-collaboration, and even part of predation.

> The essential key to collaboration is not a proscribed set of behaviors per se, but an internally felt experience of mutual caring about achieving each other's goals.

Proscribed collaborative behaviors and common goals do enhance collaboration effectiveness, but are not the essence of collaboration. They cannot substitute for collaboration. The internal felt experience of mutual caring about achieving each other's goals is far more central, reliable, and unequivocal – and unleashes a natural flow of collaborative work behaviors.

The raw power of shifting from the centrality of common goals and proscribed behaviors to an internal experience of caring about the other's goals can easily be underestimated. Mutual caring about achieving each other's goals directly leads to more collaborative behaviors and more successful results. It is more powerful than having the goals in common. It is more powerful than the most exacting and desirable set of proscribed behaviors. It makes collaboration the most powerful form of cooperation, and the ultimate source of power.

Consider this choice. Would you rather work together with people who share a goal with you, but do not care if you achieve your goal? Or would you rather work with people who care about you achieving your goal even if they do not share your goal? Which results in greater collaboration? In my experience, the latter wins every time, and produces more effective collaboration than working with people who share your goals but do not care about you achieving them.

The Global Picture:

Collaboration vs Self Interest

On the world stage collaboration plays an alluring role for the most dominant of private and public organizations as well countries. They are attracted by the potential of *Power through Collaboration* to enable them to achieve their goals. But, not all of the power players welcome the promise of *Power through Collaboration.* Some feel dread. They feel alarmed and threatened. They prefer a system based on competition and predation because they have already established dominant positions and are successful. They seek to perpetuate the prevailing system in which they have prospered. The uncertainty of a more collaborative system with new rules and principles is viewed as a threat that can reduce their control and associated wealth. Everyday local collaboration is not divorced from the influence of such powerful parties on collaborative practices. Due to the ubiquitous and infectious influence of the power players, the larger picture needs to be understood.

Some power players who see *Power through Collaboration* as a threat to their dominance and control act to hinder PtC collaboration. They undermine *Power through Collaboration* whenever they can as a matter of practice and policy. Others wield their power via an anti-collaborative overall strategy, but attempt to seize the benefits of *Power through Collaboration* at the local level or in special situations where they need it to achieve their goals. They especially value *Power through Collaboration* at the operational level. They want other people working together to more effectively, orderly, and obediently achieve predetermined plans and goals. They do not want those same people scrutinizing, much less questioning, the non-collaborative business models, strategies, or overarching goals.

Still others try to operate via a collaborative big picture strategy, but become entangled in anti-collaborative practices at the local level or for tactical expediency.

Ironically, I have experienced helping groups and organizations overcome their seemingly unresolvable conflicts and learn to collaborate with each other, only to have them view their new collaboration capability as a tool to more effectively, even if unnecessarily, do battle against others. Despite achieving what previously seemed an unobtainable level of collaboration among themselves, they resisted exploring how to collaborate with other designated adversaries. They wanted to keep their newfound *Power through Collaboration* for themselves and their own purposes.

Many seek to limit the benefits of *Power through Collaboration* to just their own group or organization. They want to use *Power through Collaboration* to achieve only their own goals. Paradoxically, *Power through Collaboration* is sometimes used to try to more effectively compete with, defeat, enslave, or prey on others.

Confining *Power through Collaboration* to an insular group can be a precursor to the paradoxical cooptation of collaboration for anti-collaborative purposes. This all too common inclination can be counteracted by using *Power through Collaboration* to engage with an expanding number of people, groups, and organizations. Best of all is building *Power through Collaboration* into the foundation and basic processes of any large-scale system.

Doesn't Self-interest Drive Achieving Goals?

Mutual caring about achieving each other's goals directly elicits reliable collaborative behavior. Nevertheless, the notion that it is more potent in enabling collaboration than a set of proscribed behaviors related to achieving common goals is deemed by some people as idealistic, moralistic, impractical, or even *nutty*. They relegate mutual caring about achieving each other's goals to the province of philosophy or religion, and as suitable only for charitable or band-aid operations for the benefit of a select or lucky few.

Many are skeptical that people will work to achieve goals that are not their own. They believe people are primarily, if not solely, motivated by self-interest. They reject explanations of human behavior not based on self-interest. They do not trust situations where they cannot point to self-interest as the explanation for people working together. They reason: "Why would someone work unless it had a direct benefit for them?"

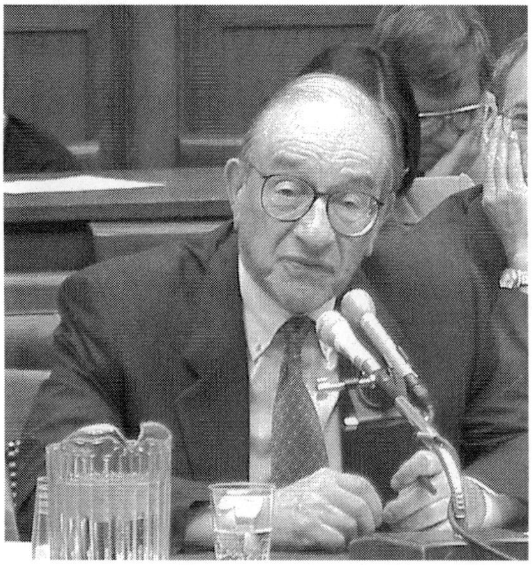

Figure 1: Alan Greenspan testifying before Congress. (Photo courtesy of Wikipedia Media Commons).

One person who apparently thought this was *Alan Greenspan*, the renowned former Chairman of the *US Federal Reserve Bank*. As Fed Chairman, and one of the most powerful people in the world, he literally *bet the bank* on the power and righteousness of self-interest and competition to function as the primary operating mechanism of a highly interdependent and complex global economic system.

That bet proved disastrous. Alan Greenspan's long and distinguished career garnering glowing praise and prestigious awards led up to, and ended with, the unfolding of the world wide Great Recession, the most severe economic crisis since the Great Depression. *Time Magazine* listed him as third out of 25 on a list of people who were most to blame for the catastrophe.

After 18 years as Federal Reserve Bank Chairman, Alan Greenspan learned an extremely painful lesson about the limits of self-interest as a basis for running an economic system:[2]

> "I found a flaw in the model that I perceived is the critical functioning structure that defines how the world works."
>
> "Those of us who have looked to the self-interest of lending institutions to protect shareholder's equity, myself especially, are in a state of shocked disbelief. Such counterparty surveillance is a central pillar of our financial market's state of balance."
>
> "I made the mistake of presuming that the self-interest of organizations,

specifically banks and others, were such that they were best capable of protecting their own shareholders and their equity in the firms."

The importance and value of self-interest in driving human behavior is impossible to deny. So is its limits, as Alan Greenspan's belated awareness attests. Other equally important drivers of human behavior are at work, and vitally needed, especially in the functioning of a complex and interdependent economic system.

Caring for Others' Goals - the Unappreciated Co-driver of the World Economy.

People willingly and often enthusiastically work toward goals other than their own, and that are beyond their own immediate self-interest. Some common reasons people can care about achieving other people's goals and be motivated to work to achieve them are family and social relationships and bonds, group membership and identification, inspirational leadership, and shared values.

Well before Alan Greenspan's painful lesson, none other than *Adam Smith*, legendary chief evangelist of self-interest driven capitalism wrote:

> "How selfish soever man may be supposed, there are evidently some principles in his nature, which interest him in the fortunes of others, and render their happiness necessary to him, though he derives nothing from it, except the pleasure of seeing it."[3]

Who at a *World Economic Forum* annual meeting was quoting Adam Smith's words? None other than *Bill Gates*, founder and Chairman of *Microsoft*, one of the richest persons in the world, and a reputed fierce business competitor. Bill Gates went on to further state,

> "As I see it, there are two great forces of human nature: self-interest, and caring for others."[4]

Self-interest is an integral aspect of human nature, and indeed, essential for survival. So is caring for others. Both are natural, and both are needed. Either operating without the other is a prescription for disaster.

The tragic Challenger and Columbia space shuttle explosions have become classic

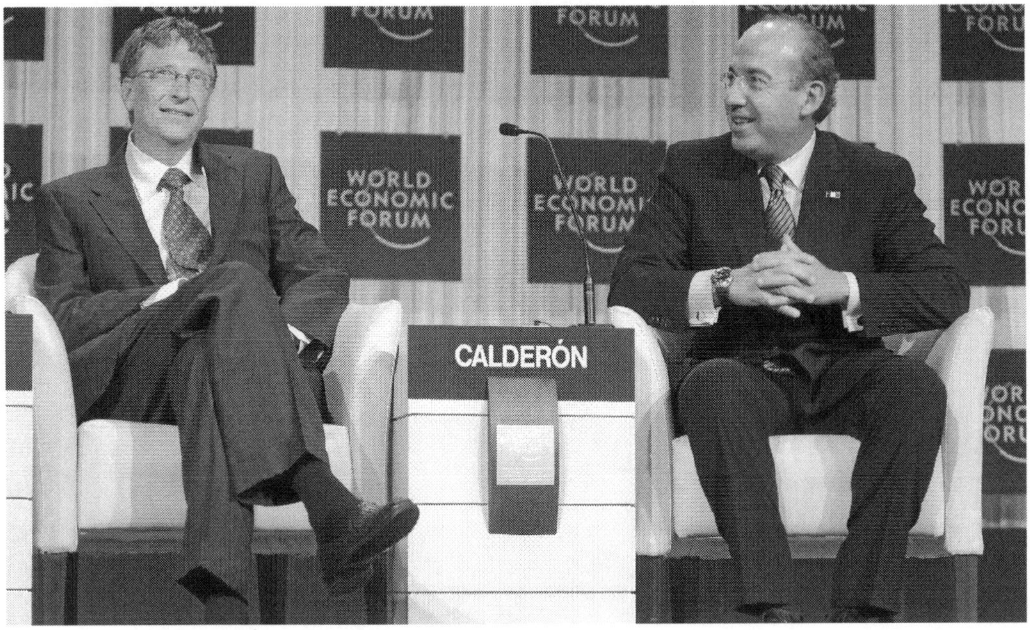

Figure 2: Bill Gates on left at World Economic Forum. (Photo courtesy of the World Economic Forum & Sebastian Derungs).

examples of disasters linked to collaboration failure. Additional examples include the mismanaged emergency response to Hurricane Katrina; the intelligence community dysfunctions related to 9/11 and the Iraq weapons of mass destruction analysis; and the actions leading up to the BP/Deepwater Horizon oil well blowout. Another epitome of catastrophic collaboration failure to add to the list is the Great Recession – a devastating collaboration failure on a colossal scale.

The Great Recession Collaboration Failure.

For the PtC Model, the Great Recession is a *massive global collaboration failure* caused by a lack of collaboration in the economic and social system, which in turn was due to operating an interdependent global economy via self-interest and competition, not only with respect to allocation of resources, but also with respect to control over the levers of political and economic power. Predatory enterprises controlled the very system safeguards intended to protect society, as well as themselves. With the predators only looking out for themselves, no one with sufficient power was looking out for the wellbeing of the system or the people in it.

James Galbraith, author of eight economic books and former Congressional Joint Economic Committee executive director, writes in his book *The Predator State*:[5]

> "The predatory class is not the whole of the wealthy; it may be opposed by many others of similar wealth. But it is the defining feature, the leading force. Its agents are in full control of the government under which we live."
>
> "Everywhere you look, the public decision is made by the agent of a private party for the purpose of delivering private gain. ... Predatory regimes ... are intrinsically unstable, something that does not trouble the predators but makes life for the ordinary business enterprise exceptionally trying."

With predators in control and no capable parties looking out for the viability of the overall economic ecosystem, the predators engorged themselves until the prey were depleted and the economic system crashed. The scenario was entirely predictable. The only mystery was when and how terrible would be the disaster. True to form, when disaster hit, the surviving predators used it to protect themselves at the further expense of the system. Those who caused the crisis used it to insure their own survival and gain more for themselves, and let others drown. Taken to an extreme, lack of collaboration can drown an entire society.

As *Peter Drucker*, legendary management guru, author of 39 books, recipient of the Presidential Medal of Freedom from President George W. Bush, and seven-time recipient of the McKinsey Award from the Harvard Business Review, put it:

> "...all earlier pluralist societies destroyed themselves because no one took care of the common good."[6]

Along similar lines, *Clive Boddy* states in the *Journal of Business Ethics:*

> "... psychopaths working in corporations, and in financial corporations in particular, have had a major part in causing the crisis. ... Corporate Psychopaths may have acted recently to the detriment of many."[7]

The Great Recession tore the veil off the delusional yet vaunted myth that prosperity lay in enabling societal control by self-interested parties pursuing their self-interest. This equates to heading for the moon by taking a submarine to the depths of the ocean. If people with power and resources are green lighted to maximize only their own interests, then they will achieve that result. Achieving prosperity for the larger community needs to include empowering people with power and resources to engage in actions that deliberately benefit the larger community.

Figure 3: Peter Drucker. (Photo courtesy of Jeff McNeill.)

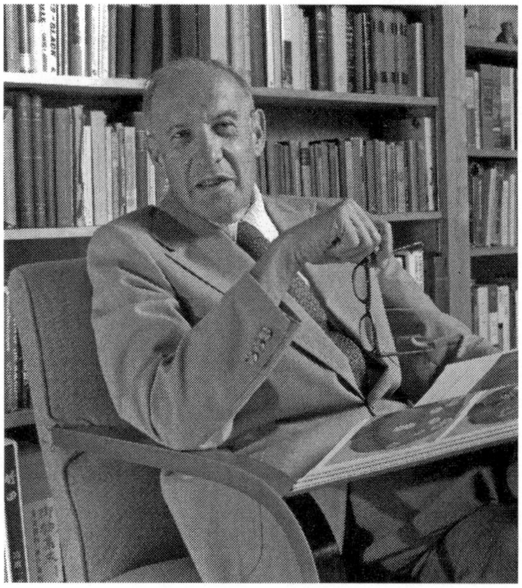

Self-interest must be taken into account, and worked with. So must caring for others. What if the global economic foundation had been built not only on self-interest, but also upon Adam Smith's other *principle of nature* and Bill Gate's other *great force of human nature*, that is, *caring for others*?

If the goal is an economy that provides widespread benefit and maximizes achievement and productivity, not doing so is as irrational as it can get. The flaws and systemic risks of basing a complex interdependent global economy on the confining dictates of self-interest are apparent not only in hindsight, but also in foresight. The disastrous results are not shocking to those who do not close their minds to incorporating that other great force of human nature, *caring for others.*

> Ignoring the power of our natural self-interest would certainly be a disastrous mistake. Just as predictably, ignoring the power of caring for others has proven to be a disastrous mistake.

Business Models Based on and Operating via Power through Collaboration.

Gary Hamel, the *Wall Street Journal's* most influential business thinker in the world, *Fortune* Magazine's *world's leading expert on business strategy*, and author of *What Matters Now*, states:

> "It's time to radically revise the deeply etched beliefs about what business is for, whose interests it serves, and how it creates value. We need a new form of capitalism for the 21st century – one dedicated to the promotion of greater wellbeing rather than the single minded pursuit of growth and profits; one that doesn't sacrifice the future for the near term; one with an appropriate regard for every stakeholder; and one that holds leaders accountable for all of the consequences of their actions.... This isn't a new challenge, but it's more urgent than ever."[8]

The Circular Economy is one such model, and is championed by the *Ellen MacArthur Foundation* and partners *B&Q*, *British Telecom*, *Cisco*, *National Grid*, *Renault*, and *McKinsey & Co.* The Circular Economy uses systems thinking to design a sustainable and restorative economic system that mimics natural living ecosystems. It rebuilds social, economic, and natural capital; operates via renewable energy; and replaces cradle-to-grave with cradle-to-cradle concepts whereby what was formerly considered waste is re-purposed as inputs for other users.[9]

Conscious Capitalism progresses along similar lines with the involvement of companies such as *The Container Store*, *Google*, *Trader Joes*, and *Whole Foods*. Conscious Capitalism businesses advocate the following:

- "a higher purpose transcending profit maximization."
- "are explicitly managed for the simultaneous benefit of all interdependent stakeholders, including customers, employees, investors, suppliers, and the larger communities in which the business participates."
- "reject a zero-sum, trade-off oriented view of business and look for creative synergistic win-win approaches that offer multiple types of value simultaneously to all stakeholders."[10]

In his book *Firms of Endearment: How World Class Companies Profit from Passion & Purpose, Raj Sisodia*, co-founder and chairman of the *Conscious Capitalism Institute*, reports that Conscious Capitalism businesses outperform by a 9 to 1

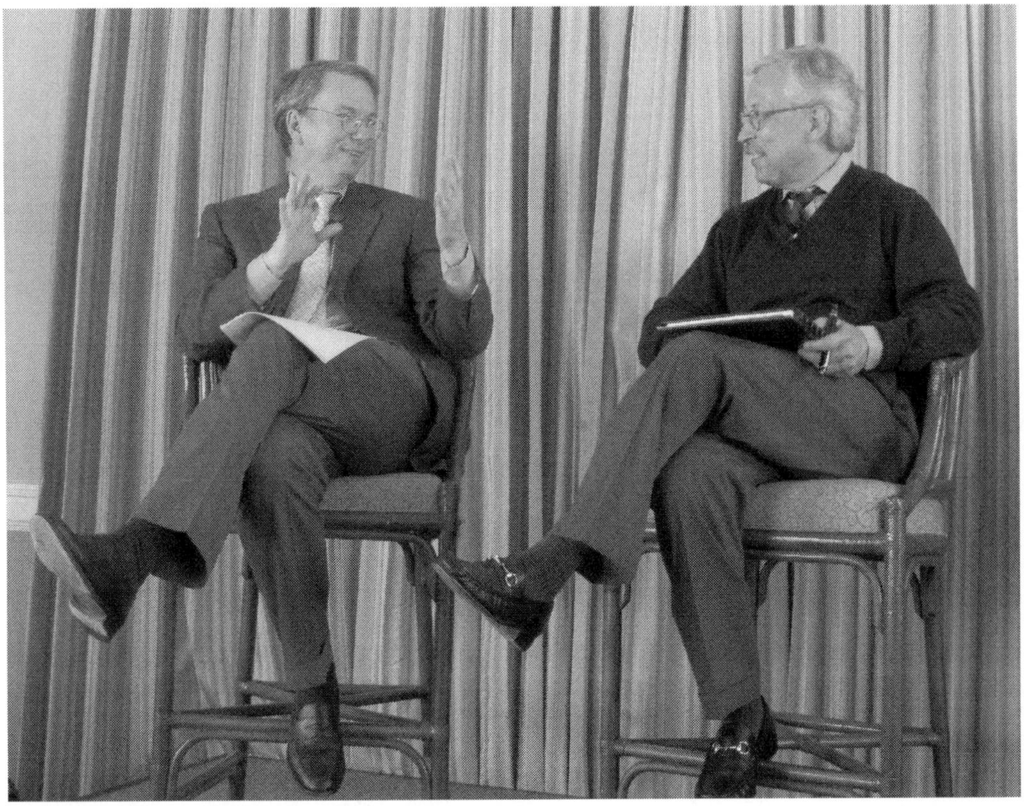

Figure 5: Gary Hamel on left interviewing Google CEO Eric Schmidt. (Photo courtesy of Steve Jurvetson).

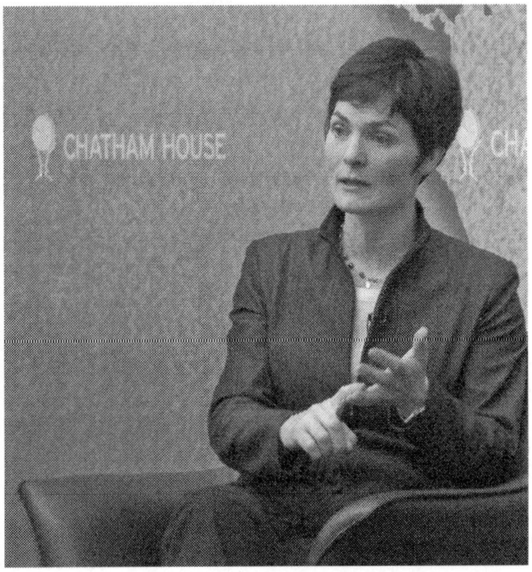

Figure 4: Dame Ellen MacArthur on Circular Economy and Redesigning the Future. (Photo Courtesy of Chatham House).

ratio, yet "pay their rank-and-file employees much better than their peers, have suppliers who are profitable, invest heavily in their communities, pay taxes at a higher rate, provide terrific customer service, invest in making their operations more environmentally sustainable and do not externalize costs onto society."[11]

Joe Keefe is President and CEO *of Pax World Management*, which manages approximately $2.5 billion in financial assets by following a sustainable investing approach. He was named by *Ethisphere Magazine* as one of the "100 Most Influential People in Business Ethics" for 2007, 2008, 2011, and 2012. In a *Green-Money Journal* interview, he advocates for Sustainable Capitalism, an economic system that:

> "… explicitly integrates environmental, social and governance (ESG) factors into strategy, the measurement of outputs and the assessment of both risks and opportunities…. The connections between economic output and ecological/societal health are no longer obscured but are expressly linked."
>
> "We will need to consistently critique the notion that externalities associated with economic output are somehow collateral, or that financial return is sufficient without beneficial societal returns, or that markets are inherently efficient and self-correcting. We will need to unabashedly offer sustainable investing not as an alternative approach but as a better approach – as the only sensible, responsible way to invest."[12]

Along a similar track, the Benefit Corporation is a relatively recent model of a state corporate charter that specifically permits corporations to take into account and serve the interests of all stakeholders, not just shareholders. The number of states that are legalizing this new corporate charter has been rapidly expanding. Additionally, a separate but aligned certification is offered by *B Labs*, which was co-founded by *Jay Coen Gilbert*, *Bart Houlahan*, and *Andrew Kassoy*. The B Lab's "Declaration of Interdependence" includes:

> "We envision a new sector of the economy which harnesses the power of private enterprise to create public benefit. This sector is comprised of a new type of corporation, the B Corporation which is purpose-driven, and creates benefit for all stakeholders, not just shareholders. … That, all business ought to be conducted as if people and place mattered; That, through their products, practices, and profits, businesses should aspire to do no harm and benefit all; To do so, requires that we act with the understanding that we are each dependent upon another and thus responsible for each other and future generations."[13]

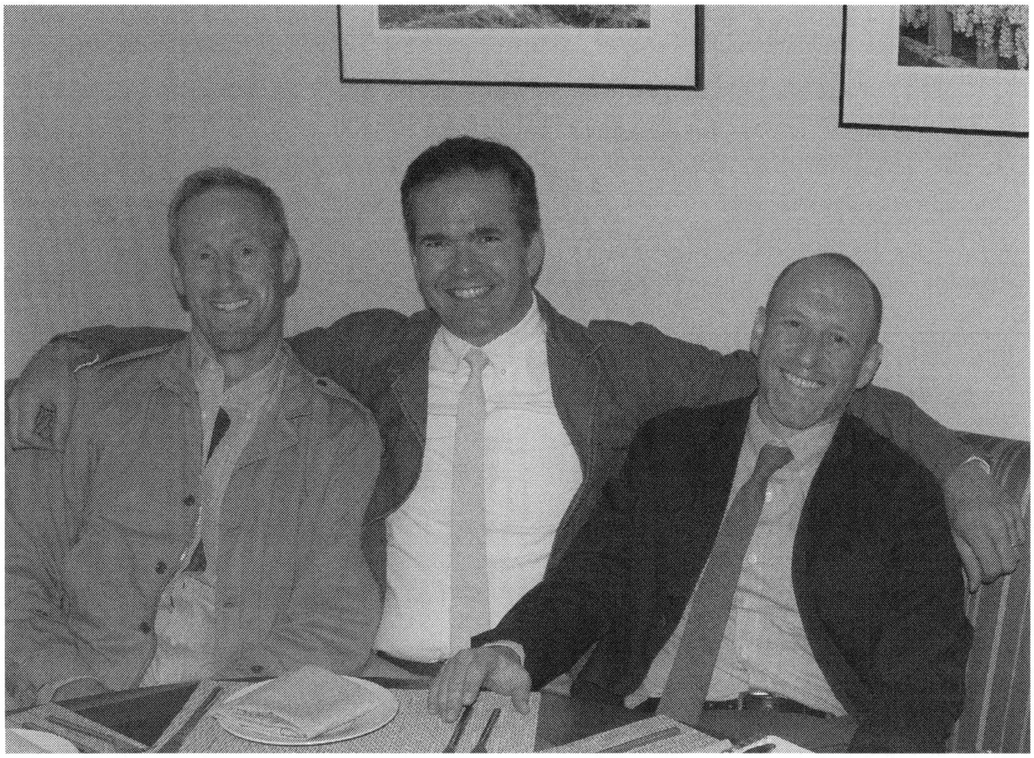

Figure 7: Co-founders of B Labs: Jay Coen Gilbert, Bart Houlahan, & Andrew Kassoy. (Photo courtesy of Andrew Kassoy).

Figure 6: Joe Keefe, CEO of Pax world Management. (Photo courtesy of Pax World.)

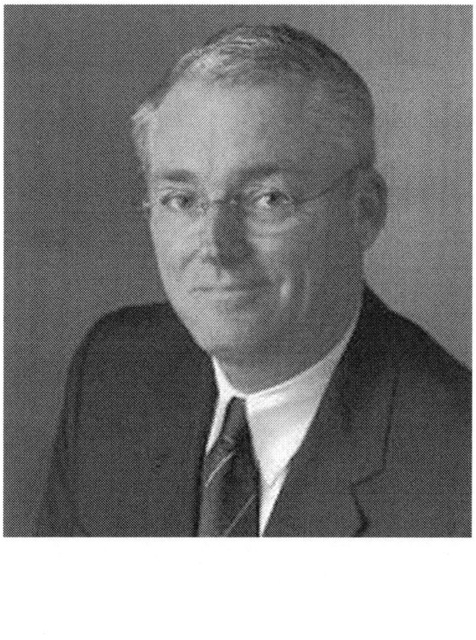

Andrew Kassoy, a B Lab co-founder, also states:

> "The private sector has become the most powerful force on the planet, dominating our social and economic lives. Therefore, we must harness the power of business to create value for society, not just for shareholders."[14]

Gary Hirschberg's business operates by similar principles. He is the founder and Chairman of *Stonyfield Farm*, the world's leading organic yogurt producer; author of *Stirring It Up: How to Make Money and Save the World*; founder of Social Venture Institute "boot camp" for community-minded entrepreneurs; recipient of numerous awards including eight honorary doctorates. His company mission includes "to serve as a model that environmentally and socially responsible businesses can also be profitable."[15] In a *Greenbiz.com* interview, Gary Hirshberg described Stoneyfield's accomplishments:

> "Much of what we set out to do at the outset was pretty much a hypothesis. The whole proposition said you can pay farmers fair prices and still make money. You can pay employees fair wages and still make money. You can use metrics to reduce your company's carbon footprint and still make money." ... "We've proven you can bake those considerations into the DNA of an enterprise and not just make money, but make more money. Our profit margin is superior to most in our segment."[16]

Factoring a social and economic mission into the business model was not a handicap, but a driver for success, and produced "a compounded annual growth rate of 27.4% over eighteen years"[17] Gary Hirshberg states in an interview with Barry Estabrook for *www.theatlantic.com* that:

> "In the end everyone wins: the farmers, the cows, the consumers, the employees, and our shareholders. ... the Stonyfield model is one any corporation can replicate, no matter how large."[18]

Also operating by similar principles is the *social business* model of *Muhammad Yunus*, author of *Building Social Business: The New Kind of Capitalism That Serves Humanity's Most Pressing Needs*, and recipient of the Nobel Prize, the Presidential Medal of Freedom, and the U.S. Congressional Gold Medal.

Whereas Alan Greenspan, as Chairman of the powerful Federal Reserve Bank, bet the world economy on the myth and delusion of the infallibility of self-interest, Dr. Yunus, as Chairman of a bank guided by *caring for others*, made the opposite bet. He founded the *Grameen Bank* with a social mission to help the poor.

Figure 9: Gary Hirshberg; (Photo courtesy of Stoneyfield Farms).

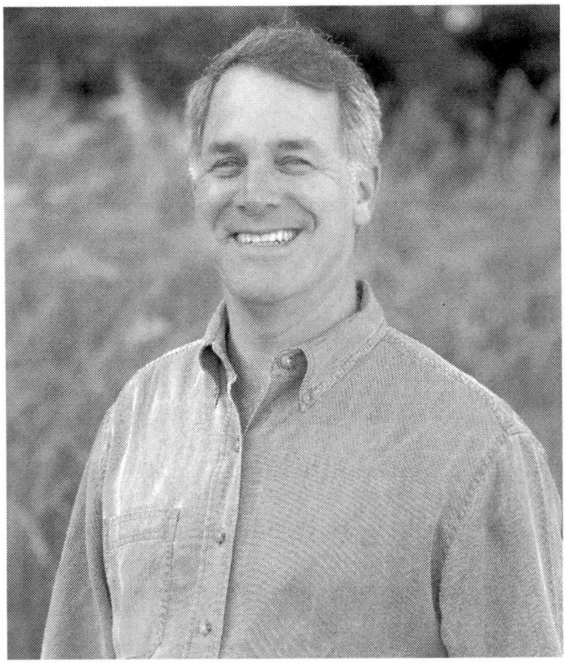

Figure 8: Muhammad Yunus. (Photo courtesy of World Economic Forum and Michael Wuertenberg).

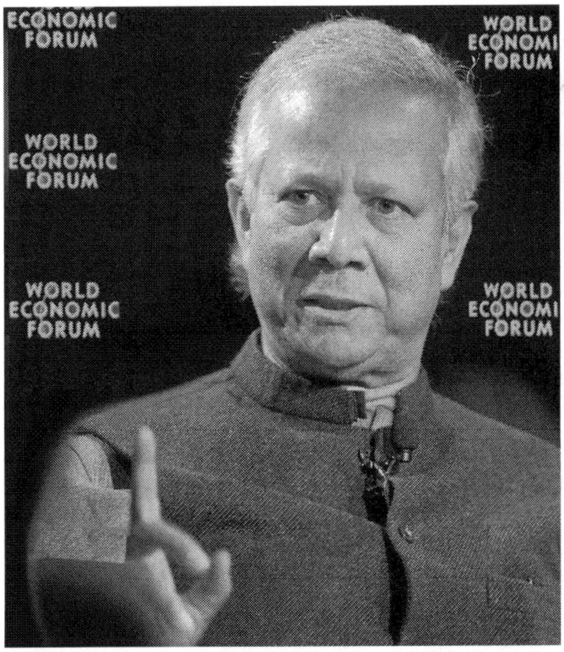

Despite its humble beginnings, Grameen Bank grew to lend almost 8 billion dollars to over seven million poor people, and is 97% owned by the borrowers, some of whom sit on the Board of Directors of the bank. Dr. Yunus started over 30 other *social businesses* including Grameen Kalyan, which operates 54 health care clinics for the poor.

Another of Dr. Yunus's social businesses was started in collaboration with *Franck Riboud*, CEO of *Groupe Danone*, a $20 billion dollar international food company. They formed a joint venture, Grameen Danone Foods Ltd, with a social business mission to reduce poverty, create jobs, and combat child malnutrition via providing a highly fortified yet affordable yogurt for Bangladeshi children.

Whereas Federal Reserve Chairman Dr. Alan Greenspan grappled with *shocked disbelief* regarding the disastrous mistake of betting the world's economic fortunes on the infallibility of self-interest, Grameen Bank Chairman Dr. Mohammed Yunus grapples with the *shock to people* who have difficulty understanding a business model based on benefiting others rather than self-interest:

> "A challenge that anyone will face in creating a social business is trying to explain why they are doing it. Our economic theories have constantly stressed that humans are self-centered beings who go about serving their own self-interest. We have been taught that as a fact for hundreds of years. Now we have an alternative, a selfless business where operators do not profit for themselves but benefit others. This can come as a shock to people. Explaining this is a challenge."[19]

> "I profoundly believe, as Grameen's experience over twenty years has shown, that personal gain is not the only possible fuel for free enterprise. Social goals can replace greed as a powerful motivational force. Social-consciousness-driven enterprises can be formidable competitors for greed-based enterprises. I believe that if we play our cards right, social-consciousness-driven enterprises can do very well in the marketplace."[20]

The Circular Economy, the Conscious Capitalism companies, the Sustainable Capitalism companies, the Benefit Corporations, the B Lab companies, the socially and environmentally conscious business of Gary Hirshberg, and the social businesses of Mohammad Yunus, all achieve success by capitalizing on *Power through Collaboration*. Moving beyond sole reliance on self-interest, and making room for mutual caring about and working willingly and freely to achieve each other's goals has been a core driver of collaborative behavior that led to highly successful outcomes.

Power through Collaboration is the Key

PtC collaboration is distinct from and more powerful than ordinary cooperation based on self-interest or common goals. It is as close as one can get to a *Holy Grail of cooperation* that enables achieving important and strongly desired goals.

Using PtC collaboration as a co-governing mechanism for the global economy would substantially increase productivity. *Power through Collaboration* is also the key to enhancing the value and usefulness of what is produced for a greater number of people and stakeholders. We already have sophisticated financial and economic models, strategies, and formulas. We have the mind-boggling reams of information and data to funnel through them. What is lacking is real collaboration.

> PtC collaboration would be a highly productive mechanism to incorporate systematically into the foundation and everyday functioning of the global economy.

Power through Collaboration is also the key to addressing the most pressing problems of our time. Whether working through the private, public, or civil society sectors, effectively dealing with complex problems such as healthcare, housing, food, water, energy, trade, and global climate change, requires *Power through Collaboration.* The knowledge and technology exists or is within reach to address such issues. The missing piece is collaboration. Lack of effective collaboration prevents deploying our knowledge and technology to their best advantage. With *Power through Collaboration* operating, the rest falls into place.

Even that most daunting of challenges – money – can be solved via collaboration. Despite claims to the contrary, in my opinion the biggest obstacle is not primarily a lack of money. It is a lack of PtC collaboration.

For example, nearly one billion people suffer chronic hunger, and millions of children die each year from lack of food.[21,22] Yet, it is estimated that 30-50 percent of food is wasted.[23] There is plenty of food produced, but it is not available to those who need it. The solution requires *Power through Collaboration.*

With respect to an example in healthcare, the *London Declaration on Neglected Tropical Diseases* has been endorsed by numerous pharmaceutical companies, the *World Bank*, *USAID*, and the *Bill and Melinda Gates Foundation*. The declaration emphasizes the essential role of collaboration:

> "But no one company, organization, or government can do it alone. With the right commitment, coordination and collaboration ... we believe that, working together, we can meet our goals by 2020 and chart a new course toward health and sustainability ..."[24]

Follow-up implementation of the *London Declaration on Neglected Tropical Diseases* reinforced the pivotal role of collaboration: "... effective collaboration is essential if the 2020 goals for NTD control and elimination are to be reached."[25]

A specific country example further bears this out:

> "The commitment and partnership between donor agencies, the Nigerian government and in-country organizations will be able to make an impact that would not have been possible without collaboration."[26]

The missing link is PtC collaboration with respect to the acquisition and deployment of financial and knowledge resources. Deploying *Power through Collaboration* requires a consciousness and willingness to advance beyond purely self-interest driven economic and social systems. Despite the reluctance of some powerful players and many obstacles, doing so promises unparalleled rewards.

At the risk of sounding overly dramatic, I will go even further. Whether or not the human species achieves *Power through Collaboration* will determine the nature of what it will mean to be human.

Game Changing Breakthrough

Periodically, pivotal developments or inventions have transformed human capability and altered the course of human evolution. Some notable examples include: primitive tools, such as clubs and spears; the use of fire; the wheel; pack animals such as horses, mules, and camels; firearms such as the musket, rifle, handgun, and machine gun; the automobile and airplane; the atomic bomb; the telephone; the radio and the television; the computer; and the internet.

To this list I add the National Security Agency's revolutionary capability to collect and store *all* internet traffic and telephone communications. The momentous significance of the ability to monitor and store the totality of today's indispensable means of communicating, interacting, and functioning is not fully appreciated by most people as they go about their everyday routines. Yet, it is at the very least on a par with previous historic breakthrough developments and inventions.

Understanding the awesome potential, the United States intelligence community is in the vanguard of deploying collaboration technologies and processes. *James Clapper*, the *Director of National Intelligence* and person responsible for oversight of all the US intelligence agencies, stated in the *Wall Street Journal*:

> "We now collaborate on intelligence collection and analysis in ways that were unheard of 10 years ago. … We now start from the imperative of 'responsibility to share,' in order to collaborate with and better support our intelligence consumers – from the White House to the foxhole."[27]

The capacity to store and analyze all internet and phone communications is a total game-changer with mind-boggling consequences. A capability upgrade of historic proportions has been attained. The NSA with its *total information awareness* program intercepts, monitors, analyzes, and stores the email, Google searches, Facebook posts, social media, telephone calls, fax transmissions, bookstore purchases, library checkouts, movie rentals, travel records, parking receipts, bank records, credit card charges, and more of whomever they choose, whenever they choose.[28]

The location and movements of people can be monitored using satellites, drones, GPS devices, radio frequency identification chips, ID cards, cell phones, and more. Video surveillance cameras are everywhere and proliferating exponentially in airports, train stations, stores, schools, workplaces, and public streets.

All of this is enabled by our breakthrough collaboration technology, which is also used in the workplace by companies to monitor and control online and offline activities of employees. Outside the workplace, personalized micro-marketing practices routinely include online and offline monitoring, and the collection and storage of massive amounts of detailed information regarding people's most intimate habits and preferences. Moreover, search engines are a major collector of our most intimate information, as John Herman describes in a *CNN Tech* article:

> "… Google knows the things you wouldn't ask your friends. It knows things you can't ask your spouse. It knows the things you haven't asked your doctor

> yet. It knows things that you can't ask anyone else and that might not have been asked at all before Google existed. Google's servers are a repository of the developed world's darkest and most heartbreaking secrets, a vast closet lined with millions of digital skeletons that, should they escape, would spare nobody."[29]

A mega-billion-dollar industry collects, organizes, correlates, stores, and with few real limits circulates our personal information far and wide. What was previously highly sensitive and private is now sold and resold to any interested buyer.[30]

Powerful groups have always sought to monitor and exert control over entire populations and societies. The day has arrived in which that capacity has scaled up to an unheard-of magnitude. The writing is on the wall. The ability to monitor and control people has reached the point where no one can escape. Not even the very people who are driving, designing, and building the technological architecture of our new connected world. It can entrap them in a suffocating web as easily as anyone else. Ironically, they risk losing the most from the system they create.

A case in point involves *General David Petraeus*, a highly decorated four-star general who served as Commander of U.S. Forces in Afghanistan, Commander of U.S. Central Command, Commanding General in Iraq, and Director of the *Central Intelligence Agency* (CIA). He dealt with collaboration technology from all angles, including being accountable for monitoring and collecting intelligence on CIA persons of interest, and for preserving CIA secrecy. Yet, collaboration technology breached his personal life and shattered his highly distinguished career.

Thousands of the general's personal emails were ensnared in an FBI investigation and revealed his extramarital affair. He was forced to resign as CIA director. Via collaboration technology, personal details and photos of the general and woman involved zoomed round the world. Gerry Smith notes in a *Huff Post Tech* article:

> "The fact that Petraeus's affair with Broadwell came to light, despite their efforts to cover it up, highlights the challenges of privacy in the digital age. 'Online privacy is hard, perhaps too hard,' Christopher Soghoian said. 'If the director of the CIA and Ms. Broadwell had backgrounds in intelligence and they couldn't keep their information private, what hope is there for the average citizen?'"[31]

The events had been set in motion by a preceding collaboration technology breach of the personal life of *General* John *Allen*, a four-star Marine Corp general whose distinguished career included the top leadership role in Afghanistan and Deputy

General David Petraeus and woman he became involved with. (Photo courtesy of US Navy).

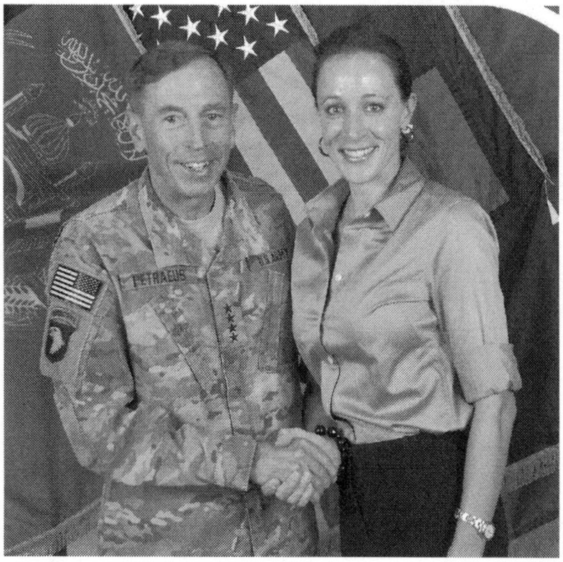

General John Allen on right in picture receiving promotion to General. (Photo courtesy of US Navy).

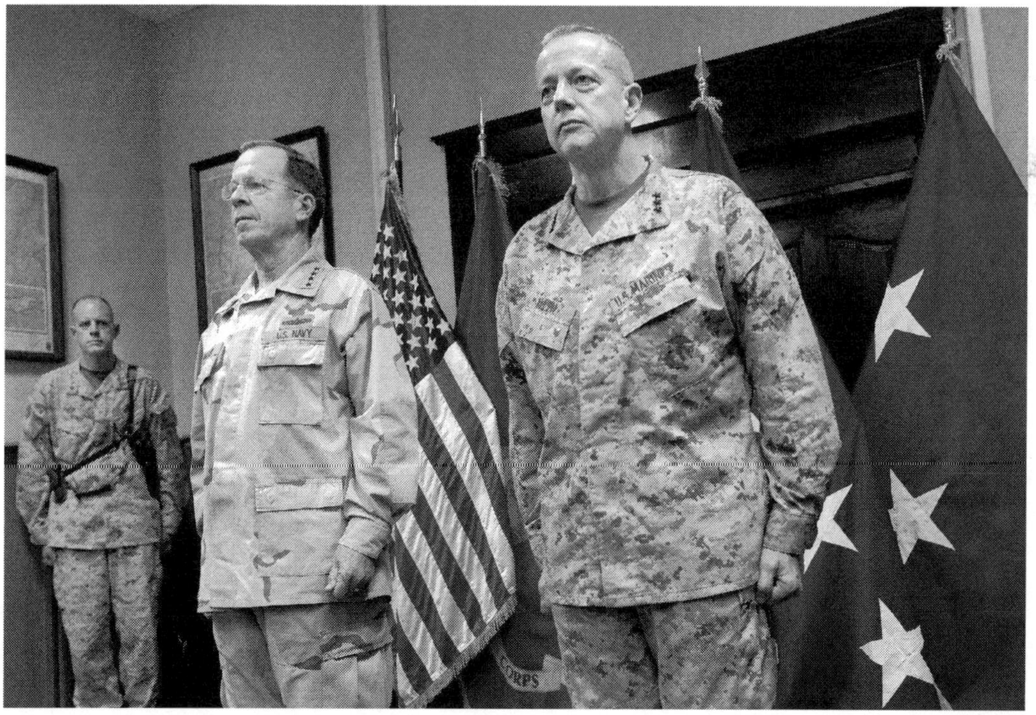

Commander of U.S Central Command. General Allen was accused of having an extramarital affair with a Tampa socialite who was viewed as a rival for General Petraeus's attention and affections by the woman General Petraeus was involved with. The woman's emails to the socialite warning her to stay away from General Petraeus triggered the FBI investigation.

Although General Allen was cleared of the allegations, the investigation probed and put into public view analysis of nearly 30,000 pages of the general's personal emails with the socialite woman in question.[32] General Allen was subsequently nominated to head the U.S. European Command and to lead all NATO forces in Europe. However, partly because of the investigation and controversy as well as health issues in the family, General Allen chose to retire instead.

> As these high profile cases demonstrate, collaboration technology and processes can be used to catch anyone and everyone in the net.

Fateful Fork in the Road

We are at a turning point for the long-term. Much is at stake. The mechanisms put in place now will shape not only our behavior in the short run, but also our basic human nature and the foundation of our social systems.

We are at a fork in the road that leads to humans becoming mere automatons subject to precise monitoring, control, and programming, whether by governments, private corporations, or powerful individuals and groups. Or becoming more highly developed, conscious, and empowered in our ability to work together. The choice will determine whether society evolves to be more collaborative or more effective at predation and enslavement. *Power through Collaboration* is essential. Without it, a fateful journey will proceed along the ominous fork in the road.

Looking at the era of Nazi rule provides some foresight regarding where such a path can lead. The Nazi regime was infamous for the efficiency of its destructive machine, which was operated in part by their then state-of-the-art computerized cooperation technology. For example, the Nazi Gestapo utilized the earliest generation of computer systems to successfully identify, target, and round up millions upon millions of so-called *undesirables*, and then efficiently transport them to a network of concentration camps.

The Nazis and the Gestapo achieved their lethal cooperation and efficiency via reliance on fear, coercion, and brutish power – not collaboration. They were no more collaborative than a lion pride hunting as a group for the next meal. They would have been most desirous and envious of the potential of our collaboration technology to aid and abet their nefarious schemes. Imagine how magnified the already enormous devastation would have been if the Nazis had our modern day collaboration tools and technology at their disposal.

Still today, some parties with certain personality types operating by certain motivations are developing and deploying collaboration technologies not to collaborate, but for the opposite ends. They seek the ironclad control and domination achieved by the Nazis. Perhaps this sounds farfetched and over-reaching?

During 40 years with the National Security Administration (NSA) and as Technical Director of its World Geopolitical and Military Analysis Reporting Group, William Binney was in the forefront of analysis and data collection of private phone calls and emails for NSA databases. This 40-year NSA veteran's view is that the United States has created a police state with few parallels in history:

> "It's better than anything that the KGB, the Stasi, or the Gestapo and the SS ever had."[33]

Such a perspective can sound extreme when applied to our reputedly democratic and free society. Perhaps it is the viewpoint of an alarmist or extremist? Who else besides a veteran NSA Technical Director could credibly assess and explain the risks inherent in our collaboration technology? The *Chairman of Google, Eric Schmidt* certainly seems like a credible source.

He shared his views in *The Dark Side of the Digital Revolution*, a *Wall Street Journal* article based on his book *The New Digital Age: Reshaping the Future of People, Nations, and Business*: [34]

> "… everything a regime would need to build an incredibly intimidating digital police state—including software that facilitates data mining and real-time

monitoring of citizens—is commercially available right now. ... and it's only logical that the configuration that one state designs (if it works) will proliferate among its allies and assorted others. Companies that sell data-mining software, surveillance cameras and other products will flaunt their work with one government to attract new business. It's the digital analog to arms sales..."

"And don't think that the data being collected by autocracies is limited to Facebook posts or Twitter comments. The most important data they will collect in the future is biometric information, which can be used to identify individuals through their unique physical and biological attributes. Fingerprints, photographs and DNA testing are all familiar biometric data types today. Indeed, future visitors to repressive countries might be surprised to find that airport security requires not just a customs form and passport check, but also a voice scan. In the future, software for voice and facial recognition will surpass all the current biometric tests in terms of accuracy and ease of use. ... With cloud computing, it takes just seconds to compare millions of faces. ... By indexing our biometric signatures, some governments will try to track our every move and word, both physically and digitally."[35]

A veritable digital arms race has been fueled by the *War on Drugs*, the *War on Terrorism*, the *War on Immigration*, and the *War on Trafficking*. Once treasured and commonly accepted privacy expectations, rights, and protections have been undermined. Enormous databases hold detailed personal information on presumed threatening people, dissenters, activists, 'persons of interest,' – and ordinary citizens. No one is exempt. Not even the architects and enablers of the new system, however clueless about this reality or its consequences some may be.

Similarly, long treasured legal protections are gone, eroded, or threatened, such as, Habeas Corpus, civil trial by peers, presumption of innocence, facing accusers and charges in court, and being informed of charges and evidence. In their place we have warrantless surveillance and secret evidence leading to unilateral, preemptive, and non-judicial restrictions, arrest, conviction, incarceration, and punishment, including summary execution.

How to make our new collaboration potential actually collaboration is an age old and universal quandary. Yet, today's *collaboration technology* has the ironic and astonishing potential to create the least collaborative scenarios imaginable.

The scary reality is at odds with the excitement around developing and deploying our new collaboration technology and tools. Collaboration 2.0 is not inherently collaborative. It is merely a tool whose potential will carve out its own inherent course and impacts on human society. We will all be swept up in collaboration technology's currents, for better or worse.

To influence the natural course that collaboration technology and processes carve out requires – genuine collaboration. It requires designing and building into the collaboration technology and tools real collaboration. It requires developing methods to actually use the tools for real and effective collaboration. A deliberate and proactive collaborative approach is needed in order to realize the empowering rather than the enslaving side of collaboration technology's awesome potential. Genuine PtC collaboration is needed as never before.

> Despite the potentially far-reaching and terrifying impacts on human freedom and self-agency, there is no going back. The technological capability has been unleashed and is only growing stronger. It already is and increasingly will be a way of life.

Making collaboration technology really collaborative as well as helping to address our most crucial issues are already enormous tasks for *Power through Collaboration.* If we do not shrink from facing the daunting risks that confront us, *Power through Collaboration* has an additional critical function. *Power through Collaboration* is an essential key to human survival.

For example, self-interest as the sole or predominate foundation of our economic system can lead to rendering the global ecosystem unfit for human life. Human impacts on climate change are leading us down an uncertain and risky path. In addition, our unprecedented destructive capability triggers the highest alert level with warning lights flashing bright red. Due to earthshattering advances in nuclear and biochemical weapons capability, the destructive consequences of human violence and war have never been greater.

Power through Collaboration is vital if we hope to avert disaster for the human species, if not the entire planet. In the larger evolutionary picture, PtC collaboration is a crucial mechanism for avoiding nuclear, bio-chemical, or climate-change self-destruction, and for shifting to a new form of power for both everyday and evolutionary survival and success.

We need to be clear about what genuine collaboration actually is and get collaboration done right. To prevent stuck, derailed, and misused collaboration technology and processes, the collaboration process needs to include specific essential components. In addition, the psychological type and motivation of the participants need to be factored into the equation. Type and motivation need to be synched up with the essential collaboration process components. People who only focus on the structure or mechanics of the collaboration process can more readily get stuck, taken advantage of, and end up with collaboration failure, possibly on a historic grand scale.

The importance of transitioning to the exertion of power based on *Power through Collaboration* cannot be overstated. It is one of the most vital and game changing quests of our time. It is essential to move beyond the fickleness and limitations of ordinary cooperation or viewing collaboration as the *standing down* or non-exertion of power. We need a formula for *Power through Collaboration* that is the psychosocial equivalent of the classic formula $e = mc^2$.

> We need a formula that enables *Power through Collaboration* to become the predominant means of exerting power, achieving success, and getting things done.

Let's look at several situations where PtC collaboration would make a decisive difference, and the people involved would love to have such a formula to reap the benefits of *Power through Collaboration*.

Examples of PtC Collaboration in Action

The PtC Model's definition of collaboration is a major shift with significant ramifications, especially for people accustomed to viewing the conduct of business as a version of warfare. Many people base their business strategies on military strategies. They view business as a cutthroat competition in which winning is everything. They question that PtC collaboration can be put into real life action. They cannot see how they could possibly care about achieving the other's goals when they are trying to defeat or destroy them.

PtC collaboration is a marked departure from business as usual. It leads to very different behaviors and opens up new vistas and alternatives. In order to illustrate how PtC collaboration influences real life behavior I will discuss it in four typical cooperation dilemmas. Names and details have been altered. Although I juxtapose *common goals* and *mutual caring about and working willingly and freely to achieve each other's goals* as if the choice was one or the other, much of the time they go together. Pulling them apart for comparison illuminates their relative power to achieve highly desired goals, as well as which is truly essential for collaboration to occur and be successful.

For each of the following four examples I have chosen several scenarios from among numerous possibilities that could be considered. Feel free to blend or revise elements of the scenarios to fit particular situations that are most relevant and of interest to you. As the presented scenarios unfold, think of how the people reacted, and how you would react if in their shoes. Think through potential options. In particular, give careful thought to how *common goals* versus *mutually caring about achieving each other's goals* would affect your decisions and behavior.

Example 1: Collaborative Partnership vs Company Breakup

Background. Jordan and a partner own a mid-sized technology company that has been very profitable and enriching for both. However, recent sales have been anemic and the company is struggling to break even. The partners expect to be able to weather the storm and are streamlining operations and preparing for eventual renewed growth.

Jordan heads up business development, and from global connections has learned of an off-the-radar game changing business opportunity. The opportunity complements and would expand current business lines, or it could also be operated as a separate enterprise, but then would compete with and undermine the existing company in some of its markets.

Jordan has a decision to make. Bring the opportunity to the current company, which would increase profitability as well as expand a core product line into new territory, and result in a significant expansion even during the current difficult period. Or alternatively, start a completely new company without the current partner, which would be more profitable freed of the current company's structural costs. The latter choice would break apart the present partnership and company.

The PtC collaboration dilemma. The pressing uncertainty is regarding what will Jordan do, and why? Will Jordan collaborate with the other partner and bring the new opportunity to the existing company? What would you do, and why?

A pivotal factor in Jordan's decision is the extent to which the partnership of the existing company is based upon cooperation and *common goals* versus collaboration and *mutual caring about and working willingly and freely to achieve each other's goals.* So, let us consider these two contrasting scenarios.

The *common goals* scenario. As a common goal, if their company gains or loses, both partners stand to financially gain or lose (stock equity and options, salary, bonuses, expense and retirement accounts, insurance policies, etcetera). If Jordan brings the new opportunity to the existing company, then both benefit. If Jordan starts a new company without the partner, then both partners lose with respect to the existing company.

If Jordan's decision is based upon the partners having common financial goals, then what would Jordan do if Jordan can gain a much better financial outcome by starting a new company without the existing partner? What happens if their common goal of financial gain diverges, or is weakened further by slumping sales, or if substantially outweighed by competing financial gains? *How much more would Jordan have to net financially before dumping the current partner and sacrificing the value of the existing company for a new company of greater value?*

The *mutual caring about and working willingly and freely to achieve each other's goals* scenario. In this scenario, the partners mutually care about and work willingly and freely to achieve each other's goals. Over years of collaborating as partners, they know, respect, and trust each other's character and values. They share important core values about the conduct and purpose of business. They feel their company mission is a manifestation of their shared values. Jordan is confident that if their situations were reversed, the partner would take into consideration and act according to what was good for Jordan as well as the partner. Both partners are accustomed to making money by working together for each other's benefit, and not just for themselves.

In this scenario Jordan mutually cares about and works willingly and freely to achieve the partner's goals. Now, *how much more would Jordan have to net financially in order to dump the current partner and sacrifice the value of the existing company for a new company of greater value?*

What would you do if you were in Jordan's situation? Would your decision be different in the *common goals* scenario than in the *mutually care about achieving each other's goals* scenario?

Example 2: Collaborative Solution Development vs Ephemeral Agreements

Background. Supporters of a wind energy project are battling opponents over where and how many wind turbines to place atop a scenic and highly visible hillside. The issue has become highly contentious, with fierce political conflict, community divisiveness, and neighbors suing neighbors.

The results of the political and legal battles to date have produced a stalemate. Neither side is able to vanquish the other. Opponents cannot completely stop construction of the wind turbines, while proponents cannot push through a maximum scale implementation. Opponents can limit the number of turbines and influence where they are sited, while proponents can construct enough wind turbines for cost effectiveness and project feasibility.

The *common goals* scenario. The battles have been time consuming, stressful, and financially draining for all involved. Given the stalemate, and little likelihood of the power balance shifting enough for one side to prevail, a common goal emerged to settle the issue with a *win-win* compromise. After all, they were all supposed to be members of the same community. Working together to achieve this common goal would save all involved considerable sums of money, stop the waste of precious community resources, end a divisive cycle of conflict, restore community civility, open the door to reconnecting, and allow everyone to get back to focusing on important community affairs.

A high profile professional collaboration process hammered out an agreement regarding the number and placement of wind turbines. Community leaders praised the agreement and emitted a collective sigh of relief that the parties had cooperated to achieve their common goal.

But wait. There is more to this story.

The <u>no</u> *mutual caring about and working willingly and freely to achieve each other's goals* scenario. Two months after the much praised win-win agreement was made, it was in tatters as the project opponents renewed the battle. Community leaders and project supporters who participated in the negotiation were left wondering what happened. They felt angry, betrayed, and baffled about what had gone wrong.

What happened was simply what often happens in *win-win* cooperative agreements driven by common goals based on convenience or necessity. Despite the common goals, the participants still only really care about achieving their own goals, and do not *mutually care about achieving each other's goals.*

Based on the materialization of the common goal of settling for a win-win agreement, participants in the negotiation cooperated. However, the parties were cooperating solely for their own interests, which happened to converge for the moment. Their common goal did not change the fact that the parties were driven to achieve only their own interests. They accepted a win-win because they got more of what they wanted than they thought they could get by continued battling or a *win-lose*. They certainly did not collaborate. They even went through a highly sophisticated process that appeared collaborative, but it was really a negotiation-taking place under a collaborative guise.

Later, the common goal based on necessity dematerialized when one faction found that they could win more of what they wanted by reneging. They no longer needed to cooperate. Therefore, they simply went ahead and reneged. When the math changed, a *win-lose* became a better deal for them than the *win-win*. They win and the other party loses. It was a simple and uncomplicated decision, and they went for it. The common goal no longer existed. They were not concerned with the other parties' goals, only their own goals. Given the opportunity, they just played a new stronger hand to get a better deal for themselves. The other side would have done likewise.

I have witnessed many highly touted, yet ostensible win-win agreements based on common goals tossed overboard in such situations! *How might this situation have played out differently if both sides mutually cared about achieving each other's goals?*

Example 3: Supply Chain Collaboration vs Supply Chain Competition

Background. Company X and Supplier M are engaged in a supply chain co-operation in which Supplier M supplies key hardware components for Company X's flagship product line. An unusually strong hurricane has disrupted operations at the Supplier M plant that manufactures the components for Company X. Flooding has put the plant out of commission for approximately four to six weeks. Only a one-week supply of components is available from inventory if Supplier M tries to fulfill the needs of all its customers, some of whom include Company X's competitors.

Company X is in a precarious position. They already have a backlog of orders to meet and are besieged with customer complaints. If Company X falls even further behind in deliveries, its stock price risks taking a considerable hit. Even more ominous is the likely hit to Company X's brand reputation, and the opportunity for competitors to increase penetration into Company X's market. If Company X does not get the inventory from Supplier M, and it goes to their main competitor, they risk losing a significant portion of their market to that competitor. If they do get the inventory from Supplier M, but pay too high a premium for it, then they will incur a loss on the sales that are already in the pipeline and paid for. In addition, increasing the price for new orders can result in customers switching to their competitors. If the situation goes badly enough, a weakened Company X could lose its market dominance for the long-term.

Company X is demanding Supplier M's entire inventory and wants priority fulfillment over Company X's competitors. Additionally, Company X wants Supplier M to honor its price commitments as contracted per previously agreed upon risk mitigation provisions, which include Company X's covering any extra costs for expedited and special handling. However, Company X's major competitor sees a serendipitous opening to capture a significant chunk of Company X's customers, and is offering Supplier M a hard-to-resist premium price for the inventory, plus a stepped-up supply chain collaboration on very favorable terms.

The PtC collaboration dilemma. Supplier M has a crucial decision to make regarding which of its customers will have top priority. The pressing dilemma is fraught with uncertainty regarding what Supplier M will do. Will Supplier M collaborate with Company X? Will it honor its supply chain contracts and deliver the necessary components to Company X at previously agreed upon pricing? Or will it have its lawyers finesse and dispute the existing contracts, and sell its inventory to Company X's competitor for a lucrative windfall profit and a new supply chain partner? What would you do, and why?

A pivotal factor in Supplier M's decision is the extent to which the supply chain collaboration with Company X is based upon routine cooperation and *common goals* versus PtC collaboration and *mutually caring about and working willingly and freely to achieve each other's goals*. So, let us consider these two contrasting scenarios.

The *common goals* scenario. As a common goal, when Company X fulfills its customers' orders, Supplier M benefits from sales of the hardware component it supplies. The greater Company X's sales are, the greater Supplier M's sales are. Both companies make more money when Company X can sell more product. And vice versa if sales decrease. The companies gain and lose in tandem.

In the hurricane crisis situation, if Supplier M supplies its inventory to Company X, both companies benefit as usual. Additionally, by forgoing the windfall profit opportunity, Supplier M plays a pivotal role in sustaining a long-term reliable customer. If Supplier M supplies its inventory to the competitor at a premium price, it makes a windfall profit. In addition, Supplier M gains a new supply chain partner on favorable contract terms leveraged from the hurricane crisis. Supplier M has a choice of working on a common goal with Company X, or working on a common goal with Company X's competitor. Alternatively, Supplier M can charge both Company X and its competitor the maximum possible premium it can extract under the circumstances.

If Supplier M's decision is based upon the supply chain partners having common financial goals, then what happens when that common goal of Company X and Supplier M is weakened or outweighed by competing financial goals? What will Supplier M do if it can gain a much better financial outcome by supplying the competitor at windfall prices, plus still charge a windfall premium for whatever inventory it did supply to Company X? *How much more would Supplier M have to net financially before making Company X's competitor its priority, and sacrificing the value of the existing supply chain collaboration with Company X for a new one with Company X's competitor.*

The *mutual caring about and working willingly and freely to achieve each other's goals* scenario. In this scenario, Company X and Supplier M mutually care about and work willingly and freely to achieve each other's goals. Over years of collaborating through good and bad economic times, they know, respect, and trust each other's leadership, business practices, and organizational cultures. They share important core values about the conduct and purpose of business, and operate in accordance with those values.

Both companies have a history with each other of meeting and keeping their contractual commitments. Their company lawyers are utilized to draw up workable contracts, not to twist them to devious advantage, find loopholes, or seize the slightest pretense to renegotiate prices or terms.

They work together to strengthen the resilience of their supply chain as well as each other's capability as partners. They work together to anticipate and plan responses to supply chain disruptions. They engage in strategic scenario and contingency planning, and have protocols for mutual access to emergency analysis and data systems.

When internal or external circumstances have impacted either company's supply chain performance, they have proactively reached out, communicated, and worked together to solve the issues. Supplier M has well-founded confidence that if it was in Company X's predicament that Company X would work together to find a mutually beneficial solution. Both companies are accustomed to factoring each other's goals into their decision making, and making money by working together with each other's benefit in mind.

In this scenario Supplier M and Company X mutually care about and work willingly and freely to achieve each other's goals. Now, *how much more would Supplier M have to net financially before making Company X's competitor its priority, and sacrificing the value of the existing supply chain collaboration with Company X for a new one with Company X's competitor?*

What would you do if you were making Supplier M's decision? Would your decision be different in the *common goals* scenario than in the *mutually care about and work willingly and freely to achieve each other's goals* scenario?

Example 4: Collaborative Executive Teams vs Power Politics

Background. Alex, the CEO of a pharmaceutical company, needs a pivotal report completed on the clinical trials of an experimental cancer treatment drug. The report will be presented to a strategic alliance debating funding mass production and distribution. Alex has been the driving force pushing the drug's development.

However, an influential group consisting of several major shareholders as well as the Board Chair is highly skeptical about the drug's prospects and wants Alex to shift the focus to their favored drugs. Thus, the company is being rocked by open conflict and backdoor intrigue. If the report is not completed and approved by the end of the fiscal year, the opposing group could likely persuade the strategic alliance to move on to their favored drug opportunities.

The report requires the approval and analysis of Chris, EVP and Head of R&D. Alex desperately needs Chris's support. However, Chris is subject to intense pressure and not so subtle threats from other powerful people who want the drug's development quashed regardless of its merits. They are pressuring Chris to criticize and reject the drug, or at least to delay reporting the findings. Chris is just as enmeshed in the politics at the top as Alex is, and faces a fateful risk/reward and survival calculation separate from Alex's.

This example relates to the challenge of high stakes high risk collaboration versus cooperation at the top of organizations that are rocked by the intrigue and battles of powerful opponents. Whether Chris will *collaborate* with Alex depends on whether their relationship is based on the *common goals* of ordinary cooperation versus genuine collaboration and *mutual caring about and working willingly and freely to achieve each other's goals*. To illustrate what Chris might do, and why, let us look at three contrasting scenarios.

The *common goals* scenario. In this scenario, Chris's interests are aligned with Alex's interests. As key players on the executive team, they are highly visible, and squarely in the target crosshairs. Both their careers are on the line, including risk of immediate termination if matters go badly enough. Success or failure of the experimental cancer drug will decisively impact their careers, as well as their year-end stock options and bonuses.

In addition, a victory for Alex would consolidate Alex's position and power in the company as well as the strategic alliance, and greatly expand the R&D budget under Alex's control. Alex would select the person to head up the next phase of development - which could be Chris.

The *common goal*, but <u>no</u> *mutual caring about and working willingly and freely to achieve each other's goals* scenario. Consider the above common goal scenario with an added twist of Alex and Chris *not* having any mutual caring about and working willingly and freely to achieve each other's goals. In this scenario, Chris feels the job does not contribute to anything that matters to Chris. On top of that, Chris sees Alex as only concerned about Alex's career and willing to do whatever it takes to advance Alex's finances and power, even if it harms Chris. Chris is particularly upset about being in the liability hot seat as R&D chief because of Alex's garnering big bonuses by pushing poor quality drugs of questionable effectiveness and with excessive health risks. And the resultant product recalls are blamed on Chris.

Despite not caring about achieving Alex's goals, Chris has prospered financially by cooperating and going along with Alex, and still has much to gain or lose in terms of career advancement and survival, as well as immediate financial incentives. Even though Chris is not feeling good about Alex or the company, Chris still confronts the same consequences as Alex.

The <u>no</u> *common goal*, but with *mutual caring about and working willingly and freely to achieve each other's goals* scenario. In this scenario, Chris is already scheduled to retire, and will be gone and out of sight before any negative fallout with respect to the report hits. Chris has little to gain or lose whether or not the report is supportive of Alex or even done. Chris and Alex no longer have common interests and goals.

However, Chris feels mutual caring about achieving each other's goals. Chris takes the job of R&D chief very seriously, having chosen the career partly because Chris's partner had died from cancer. In addition, Chris views Alex as sharing core values, and as being a conscientious person who is passionate about getting effective and safe drugs approved and into the market place for the patients who need them.

A range of options. Alex desperately needs *Power through Collaboration* with Chris. However, collaboration, much less cooperation, is far from assured. Chris is subject to pressures counteracting those that Alex can bring to bear. Although common goals typically generate some level of cooperation, the pressures and risk confronting Chris could offset that.

Chris has many choices regarding what actions to take. The options range from collaboration to sidestepping involvement to outright sabotage. Chris has the choice to: engage in total collaboration with Alex and do the best report possible; make an effort on the report that is sufficient to protect Chris even if it does not meet Alex's needs; make excuses and shrug off responsibility leaving Alex to go it alone; focus on political maneuvering and cater to whomever appears to be holding the winning hand; work to achieve the goals of whomever will pay the most; construct a report that sabotages Alex's goals; or work to undermine Alex and get Alex fired!

With Chris's options having such disparate yet pivotal impacts, the scenario that is operating is decisive. If you were in Alex's situation, which of the above contrasting scenarios would you like to have operating? To what extent would you want Chris to mutually care about and work willingly and freely to achieve each other's goals? Which of these scenarios would provide the most powerful fuel for *Power through Collaboration* and thus would enable Alex to be able to count on the much needed backing and collaboration from Chris?

If you were in Chris's situation, which contrasting scenario would motivate you to collaborate the most with Alex? Which would motivate you to collaborate the least?

Conclusion

The preceding examples illustrate *Power through Collaboration* in operation, and lay out the very different paths taken and outcomes achieved. The range of available options and the likely behaviors are very different when operating via common goals as compared to PtC collaboration. Especially when the situation is highly challenging, such as during a crisis or when the stakes are high or the goals are crucial to accomplish, the relative power of real collaboration versus common goals is revealed. All four examples involve fateful decisions and crucial actions that require *Power through Collaboration* in order to achieve the best outcome. *Power through Collaboration* offers a significant advantage over engaging in *business cooperation as usual based primarily on common goals.*

In Example 1, whether or not a successful and still viable company can continue to survive and prosper is clouded by uncertainty. The outcome depends upon whether or not the partners *mutually care about and work willingly and freely to achieve each other's goals.*

In Example 2, regardless of what pseudo collaborative process is used, as long as the project proponents and their opponents do not *mutually care about and work willingly and freely to achieve each other's goals*, their agreements will remain fragile and liable to shift with the prevailing winds of power.

In Example 3, Company X's prospects or even survival depend upon whether its supply chain collaboration with Supplier M is truly collaborative, or based on just common goals that are being challenged by the competing goals created by the hurricane crisis. If their supply chain collaboration is based on *mutually caring about and working willingly and freely to achieve each other's goals*, then Company X can better obtain the collaboration it desperately needs from Supplier M to ward off its competitors, maintain its dominant market position, and survive.

In Example 4, if Alex and Chris *mutually care about and work willingly and freely to achieve each other's goals,* then CEO Alex can obtain the desperately needed power and benefits of collaboration in order to achieve high stakes goals in a very challenging, politically contentious, and high-risk situation.

Most if not all of the parties in these examples would love to have a formula to help them achieve the *Power through Collaboration* needed to accomplish their goals.

PtC = (T + M) x CE

Power through Collaboration

= (PtC Type + PtC Motivation)

x Collaboration Essentials

The PtC Formula

The Formula for Transforming PtC Collaboration into Power through Collaboration

PtC collaboration is valuable and needed. What is needed most is PtC collaboration that is an effective means of exerting power – the power to get things done, to achieve crucial high stakes goals, and to get outstanding results even in challenging situations. That is, what is needed most is Power through Collaboration.

So, can we reliably produce such powerful collaboration? And if so, how? Some who question the idea of collaboration being a powerful force may be inclined to dismiss the PtC definition of collaboration as an intangible, fuzzy, or unworkable concept. Or as a nice idea for a utopian realm. Or as just too complex. People related issues are often viewed as not being subject to rational formulation, rigorous analysis, and strategic implementation.

PtC collaboration and Power through Collaboration are not *aerie-fairy* concepts. They are tangible, reliable, and able to be implemented. The definition of PtC collaboration derives from psychological components that can be readily specified and integrated into a practical and usable formula for achieving Power through Collaboration. Power through Collaboration can be systematized and operationalized via the PtC Formula shown on the opposite page. The formula makes PtC collaboration powerful enough to function as Power through Collaboration.

The concrete components for constructing the PtC Formula include the psychosocial typology with respect to cooperation of the people, groups, or organizations involved; the motivations that drive them; plus the essential collaboration process components operating in the situation. These PtC Types, PtC Motivations, and Collaboration Essentials process components are specifiable and can be combined to generate the PtC Formula that produces Power through Collaboration.

The 5 PtC Types:

- Collaborator
- Cooperator
- Competitor
- Enslaver
- Predator

PtC Types

The PtC Types framework categorizes people, groups, and organizations according to their potential capability to commit to, perform effectively, and achieve goals via collaboration. PtC Type is a significant factor in determining whether investing in collaboration will pay off. Some types are better to collaborate with, and some types are better *not* to collaborate with. When considering with whom to engage in collaboration, neglecting to ascertain PtC Type can result in wasting precious time and energy. Or worse. With some types, collaboration can be not just unproductive, but even outright dangerous.

The PtC Types bring their predispositions to any cooperative endeavor, along with accompanying mindset and habitual behaviors. Pressured and stressful situations accentuate the PtC Types predispositions, bringing out the best in Collaborators or the worst in Predators, for example.

It would be great if all types were suitable for collaboration, but some just are not. Confronting the reality that some people are not capable of collaboration can be unpleasant and difficult. However, the reality that some types of people are too risky to collaborate with is one of the most important and yet most neglected factors for successful collaboration.

Clients seem to readily grasp a sense of what the PtC Type labels mean, and have been able to use the labels to communicate and work on the related issues. Although the PtC Type labels were selected in order to be self-explanatory, the specific meanings are as follows.

Collaborators: strongly value achieving the goals of both themselves and those with whom they collaborate. They prefer to collaborate and seek out collaborative opportunities. They try to maximize collaboration in cooperative endeavors. They try to make collaboration work even when it appears challenging.

Collaborator types enjoy sharing their successes with others. They appreciate the contributions of others, are sincerely generous with acknowledgement and praise, and share the limelight and credit. Highlighting and including other contributors makes the success more satisfying. Even when not directly involved, Collaborator types find satisfaction in the successes of others. They are not threatened by, but instead acknowledge and admire the talents, strengths, and abilities of others.

Collaborator types usually do not take pleasure in other's losses and disappointments, even if directly or inadvertently benefiting. If they must achieve their goals at another's expense, they see it as taking away from the success. The mutual achievement of goals is preferred as a greater and more desirable success.

When Collaborator types engage in competitive enterprises, such as business competition, sports, or games, they prefer and advocate for *fair competition* with an accompanying mindset of *may the best person, company, or team win*. They *play fair* and demonstrate basic integrity. They also prefer setting up a system in which there can be more than one winner, and in which the rewards of victory can be shared by more than one winning party.

When victorious, Collaborator types naturally take satisfaction and pride in their accomplishment and victory, but without gloating. They do not feel a need to denigrate their failed opponents. They are able to recognize the worthy abilities and performances of their competitors. They even accord due respect and offer sincere praise for the efforts of others. They are concerned about and consider ways to help the losers deal with or mitigate the consequences of losing.

Even if losing, Collaborator types can still respect people against whom they compete. Losing is disappointing, yet they still can admire the abilities and superior performance of competitors and not feel personally denigrated or inferior.

Whether winning or losing, Collaborator types can enjoy camaraderie among competitors. They can bond with competitors as fellow participants in a mutually interesting and exciting competitive arena. They contribute to making the overall structure and functioning of the competitive endeavor a collaborative one. When possible, they go beyond fair competition and promote *collaborative competition*.

Cooperators: strongly value achieving goals via cooperation and with a minimum of conflict and tension. They seek to avoid *blowback* and collateral damage from conflict. They seek out, create, and try to maximize cooperative endeavors. They try to make cooperation work even when it appears challenging. Cooperator types are open to and agreeable to collaborating provided it meets their needs.

Cooperator types are willing to share successes with others as a matter of good diplomacy. Acknowledging other's contributions avoids fallout from excluding them. Recognizing other's talents, strengths, and abilities is a pragmatic means to create goodwill. It can be useful in garnering further cooperation and success.

When engaged in competitive endeavors, Cooperator types emphasize the need to abide by the rules and regulations of *fair competition*. They behave similarly to Collaborator types, albeit with less conviction or commitment. Their encouragement of friendly competition is motivated by a concern that the tensions of competition can get out of hand and *upset the entire apple cart*. They especially want to avoid exacerbating conflict to the point where it leads to outright battle.

When victorious Cooperator types are careful not to rub it in their opponent's faces. They are concerned when others lose and worry that they may react counterproductively. They are solicitous, and attempt to mitigate ill will and avoid conflict. They are publicly diplomatic, while tactfully saving for a private audience any boastful satisfaction or negative feelings about their opponents. Similarly for the times when they are on the losing end. Cooperator types try to maintain a public composure while only sharing behind closed doors any expressions of frustration or anger.

Competitors: value winning at another's expense. They prefer to compete rather than cooperate, much less to collaborate. They seek out competitive situations. When competing they consider *fair play* to be for saps and fools. Rules are manipulated to advantage or broken whenever necessary. They do whatever it takes to win, including cheating, stealing, bribing, and sabotaging.

Competitor types do not behave much better in a cooperative endeavor. They distrust cooperation and need to be persuaded of its benefits for themselves in order to cooperate. If they engage in a cooperation endeavor, they bolt at the slightest pretense. If they stay engaged, they do not play well with others. Rather, they are preoccupied and intent on prevailing over the others. Instead of reciprocating cooperation in response to cooperation, they are constantly looking to gain some advantage from the other party's cooperative behavior. Without even trying, they can reflexively spoil cooperation situations and twist them into competitive ones.

Competitor types measure success by defeating or gaining more than someone else, rather than by normative standards. No matter how positive the feedback from others, they only feel successful if they are outdoing someone. They prefer *winner take all* competitions in which they do not have to share the rewards of victory. They do not like sharing success, hog the limelight, and take all the credit. They cut others out of the picture who may be perceived as having contributed. Competitor types are vain and gloating when successful. They denigrate and can be publicly offensive and abusive toward losing parties.

Competitor types have an especially difficult time coping with losing. They react by feeling personally deflated and inferior. They become resentful and vindictive. They disparage their opponents and undermine the merits of another's victory over them as a matter of course. They are not capable of acknowledging or appreciating, much less praising, the abilities or superior performance of other competitors. There is no getting along with other competitors. Opponents are considered enemies who must be defeated at all costs.

Competitor types find it hard to respect a worthy opponent, especially one who has defeated them. The talents, strengths, and abilities of others elicit at best begrudging acknowledgement, and ready resentment. They resent the successes of others even if they suffer no related loss or are not even involved in the situation. Just knowing or seeing others win or do well arouses envy and ill will. They take satisfaction in other's losing, and feel someone else's loss is their gain.

Enslavers: value controlling others for their own physical, financial, or emotional gain or survival. They are most comfortable with and seek out opportunities to control others to serve their needs. They have little interest in collaboration or cooperation, unless it increases their control. They readily engage in a charade of cooperation to achieve their own ends. They are always probing, maneuvering, and doing whatever is necessary to increase their control. If advantageous, they will promote the appearance of cooperation, or let others think that the others are in control. Cooperation is just another way to gain and expand control over others.

Similarly, competition is also just another process by which they gain control over others. If advantageous, they will take on the public role of being in charge or of being the winner. Letting others feel like or look like they are in charge or are the winners also works for the Enslaver type. Whatever works is fine. The only rules that matter are the ones they make and can force others to follow. Concepts of *fair play* or *foul play* are irrelevant. Whether they win or lose is irrelevant. What counts is whether they gain or lose control.

In victory and in defeat Enslavers will credit others and share the limelight, or grab it for themselves – whichever increases their control. They can be laudatory to others and self-deprecating if it gets them what they want. They can be insulting to others and self-aggrandizing if it gets them what they want. It is all about public relations and manipulation in service to their goals. Regardless of how they feel about their own capabilities, or how they stack up against other's capabilities, their primary concern is about the strategic impact on increasing their control.

Enslaver types view the capabilities and successes of others with apprehension. They are threatened by the talents, strengths, and abilities of others, and mark capable people for monitoring and extra attempts to control. The increased capability or good fortune of others is viewed as an obstacle to the Enslaver type's goals. Capable and successful people are usually harder to subdue and more troublesome to control. Enslaver types want their victims to be powerless and demoralized, or no more capable than necessary to serve their needs while still being controllable.

Predators: focus on their physical, financial, or emotional gain and survival at the expense of their prey's physical, financial, or emotional survival. They are primarily focused on their own needs and goals. They do consider the impact of their actions on others, but out of concern for themselves. They want to make sure they are not exposed and at risk, or needing to adjust their tactics. They have little interest or desire in genuinely collaborating or cooperating. They are more comfortable with and seek out predatory opportunities. For Predators, anything goes. There are no rules, except the ultimate of rules – *eat or be eaten.*

However, Predator types do cooperate, particularly if their survival requires it, or if they are getting what they want. Predator types like being fed or getting what they want without having to hunt and fight for it. Otherwise, engaging in cooperation or collaboration for the Predator type is actually part of a sophisticated hunting routine during which they camouflage themselves; hide their intentions; adjust to their prey's activities; stay on track; surreptitiously probe for weakness; and await an opportunity to strike. Meanwhile, if the other parties are lulled into believing that the Predator type is cooperating, so much the better.

Predator types prefer the shadows and avoid the limelight. They do not want to invite scrutiny. They are content to let others get all the attention. They routinely participate in praising and celebrating the capabilities and successes of others as part of their camouflage, and to catch prey off guard. If Predator types do get attention, they attempt to portray a reassuring and nonthreatening image.

On the other hand, Predator types do scrutinize others. They pay close attention to other's abilities and successes, but not to cooperate. They are looking for predatory opportunities; assessing whom to target; assessing their prey's strengths and weaknesses; taking stock of potential obstacles; and deciding when to strike. Capable prey just make their work harder, so Predator types want to determine who is the easiest prey to go after first. Capable and successful people are viewed merely as future prey that are not immediately targetable.

The 9 PtC Motivations for Cooperation:

- Survival
- External Accountability
- Internal Accountability
- Joint Defense
- Achieve Own Goals
- Common Goals
- Family and Social Bonds
- Shared Mission
- Shared Values

PtC Motivations for Cooperation

Motivation drives us to take action and achieve our goals. Motivation pushes us to act in one way rather than another. Everything that we do is driven by one type of motivation or another, and differing types of motivations drive different behaviors. So it also is with collaborative and cooperative behavior. Motivation drives collaborative behavior. Motivation drives cooperative behavior. Motivation drives non-collaborative and non-cooperative behavior. Certain types of motivation to a greater or lesser degree drive collaborative behavior, while other types of motivation to a greater or lesser degree drive non-collaborative behavior. Thus, the Power through Collaboration formula incorporates the 9 PtC Motivations for Cooperation:

The PtC Motivations for Cooperation are shown on the opposite page, and are ordered along a continuum according to how strongly they promote collaboration. Survival motivation promotes collaboration the least and Shared Values motivation promotes collaboration the most.

The PtC Motivations for Cooperation are not the usual reasons for collaboration associated with common goals, strategy, operations, business fundamentals, or risk management. Or synergies regarding products and services; brand recognition and appeal; patents and licenses; technological or production capabilities; product development and distribution channels; customer base and market dominance; capital requirements; cost effective resource utilization; etcetera.

These standard motivations for cooperation are rarely sufficient to insure collaboration success. PtC Motivations for Cooperation need to be considered, and are an essential complement to the standard motivations. Overlooking the psychological motivational framework sinks many a collaboration endeavor.

Survival. Survival motivation involves being driven by financial, social, emotional, or physical survival concerns. For example, cooperating with coworkers or supervisors to lay off other co-workers instead of oneself. Also, signing a contract with unfavorable terms because it is the only way to get what you need. Also, cooperating to keep a job you dislike but need because of financial desperation.

Survival motivation is frequently touted as a galvanizer of cooperation. It is also considered an instigator of *dog eat dog* behavior. Which is it? The answer depends on the situation as well as the PtC Type, and is discussed further in the comprehensive and advanced PtC resource book *"Power through Collaboration: When to Collaborate, Negotiate, or Dominate!"* In general, when Survival is the primary PtC Motivation, the result is usually *everyone for themself.*

External Accountability. External Accountability motivation involves being compelled by or being accountable to an outside third party subject to punitive consequences for failure to comply. For example, being ordered by a court to implement safety practices subject to a substantial fine for failure to comply. Also, being required to report to a parole officer in order to remain out of jail.

Internal Accountability. Internal Accountability motivation involves being compelled by or being accountable to a third party that one is associated with subject to punitive consequences for failure to comply. For example, an employer pressuring a salesperson to cooperate with a particularly obnoxious and difficult prospect. Also, a Board Chair may expect a CEO to cooperate with an antagonistic Board member who has the inside track on a desirable acquisition. Also, a parent might compel a child to cooperate on a project with classmates.

Internal Accountability motivation generally does not require as much pressure or persuasion as External Accountability does. Some motivated by Internal Accountability may not want to comply at all, but others may just be somewhat reluctant.

Coercion from parties that a person is associated with tends to carry less sting than coercion from outside parties. It still is prone to elicit resistance. People can agree with the need to comply but still rankle at being pushed or held accountable.

Joint Defense. Joint Defense motivation involves being driven by financial, social, mental, emotional, or physical self-defense concerns. An example is two competing companies cooperating in a lawsuit against another company that is violating their intellectual property rights. Also, two opposing political parties or groups cooperating to defeat legislation that would have negative consequences for their separate interests.

In order to draw a clear distinction, the above examples depict the parties as competitors. The parties can just as easily be friends or allies. The key point is that the parties are being driven by their own individual defense needs, which can result in a joint defense benefit. Although there may be some common interests that are protected as a by-product, Joint Defense is actually about each party cooperating with the other in order to better protect their own individual interests.

Achieve Own Goals. Achieve Own Goals motivation involves being driven to achieve one's own goals and interests. For example, working in order to get paid, have food and a place to live, or earn a promotion. Also, offering appealing benefits to retain key employees. Also, lobbying for a law favorable to one's goals. Also, joining a strategic alliance to gain market access.

Achieve Own Goals motivation can sometimes appear to produce more cooperation than is actually the case. Parties working together to better achieve their own individual goals can appear to be pursuing common goals. What often looks like the achievement of common goals is just the incidental and simultaneous achievement of the same individual goals, or a by-product of working with others to better achieve individual goals.

Achieve Own Goals motivation is often a complement to Common Goals motivation, but not vice versa. Parties who share common goals usually also have their own individual goals as well. Parties who have their own individual goals often do not share any common goals.

Common Goals. Common Goals motivation involves being driven to achieve shared goals with specific intent and not merely as a byproduct or coincidence. For example, a company and employees with a common goal of minimizing layoffs create a job-sharing program. Also, several companies that specialize in the production of different components of a new product share a common goal of making the product successful, and cooperate to do so.

Also, an employee and a company who both share an interest in each other's success cooperate on the common goal of closing a high dollar sale. If this example were an Achieve Own Goals motivation, the employee would not have the goal of increasing the company's success, and the company would not have the goal of increasing the employee's success. Each would be working to achieve only their own goals, which may or may not coincidentally end up benefitting both. The significance of this distinction is often underestimated or obscured by pressing circumstances, and only becomes salient upon achievement of the goals and the resulting difficulty divvying up the rewards.

Common Goals need to be assessed in balance with competing goals, both with regard to their number and strength. One very important competing goal can outweigh and override a host of common goals. Or a constellation of smaller competing goals can combine to impact a larger common goal.

When discussing the popular misconceptions regarding collaboration I emphasized that common goals are not the essence of collaboration. Common goals are still very much a typical and valuable part of most collaborations. They also do promote collaboration, even if they are not the essence. The preceding PtC Motivations, from Survival motivation through Achieve Own Goals motivation, can be perfectly adequate for promoting cooperation, but are generally weak at promoting collaboration. The PtC Motivations from Common Goals through Shared Values are much more potent for promoting collaboration. While not as potent as Shared Values, Common Goals motivation is the starting point at which the PtC Motivations become more capable of promoting collaboration.

Family and Social Bonds. Family and Social Bonds motivation involves being driven by a bond or association with a family or social group. For example, a union member who does not want to strike or picket doing so because of being a union member. Also, an executive considering a business proposition because it is from a member of a shared political group, country club, or fraternity/sorority. Also, a business owner hiring a family member who is not qualified.

At first glance, family bonds can seem more motivating than social group bonds. However, either can be more motivating than the other, depending upon the specific circumstances and personalities involved. Family bonds have the advantage of creating a connection from birth, but are non-elective. Social bonds may be shorter in duration and lacking *blood ties*, but are elected for a deliberate purpose.

Shared Mission. Shared Mission motivation involves being driven not just by common goals, but also by the shared core purpose of an endeavor or organization. For example, employees of a government agency and a private company valuing their mission to launch space probes. Also, an environmental organization, a public energy authority, and a private company strongly believing in the value of a renewable energy project that will fulfill their respective missions.

Shared Values. Shared Values motivation involves being driven by shared core beliefs, values, and philosophies about the purpose of work, relationships, or life. For example, the employees of an internet company believe in net neutrality and open access, and feel their company shares and advances those values through its services. Also, two companies in a joint venture feel each shares core beliefs and values about the conduct of business with customers and employees. Also, a nonprofit group feels their values as well as mission are shared by a pharmaceutical company developing a drug for an intractable disease targeted by the group.

Just as with Common Goals motivation, Shared Values motivation needs to be assessed in balance with competing values, both with regard to number and strength. One very important competing value can outweigh and override a host of shared values.

PtC Motivation Profiles. In any given situation multiple PtC Motivations of varying intensities are usually operating, and form PtC Motivation Profiles. Motivation Profiles are far from static, and can change substantially and abruptly.

PtC Motivation Profiles are unstable because which motivations are operating at what intensity can vary considerably from situation to situation. Both the particular operating motivations and their intensities can readily shift. In reaction to external events or internal personal changes, different motivations of fluctuating intensity can operate simultaneously, sequentially, or in oscillation.

People often engage in more than one cooperation situation at a time, and can operate via very different Motivation Profiles in each of them. The operating motivations and intensities of one current situation cannot be assumed to be operating also in other current situations. Similarly, past operating motivations and intensities are a guide, but not a guarantee as to which motivations will operate at what intensity in a new situation. Previous operating motivations can become inactive, while new ones become active.

Inactive motivations have the potential to be activated, thereby changing the operating Motivation Profile, and the prospects for effective collaboration. Influencing which motivations are operating in a Motivation Profile is a valid and key strategy for enhancing Collaboration Potential. For example, activating Shared Values to replace Achieve Own Goals as a primary operating motivation can substantially improve Collaboration Potential and collaboration prospects.

> Whereas PtC Types encompass stable core motivations that are an integral part of personality and that typically operate across different situations, PtC Motivations are situation specific.

The 6 Collaboration Essentials are:

- Communication
- Understanding
- Competence
- Respect
- Trust
- Safety

Collaboration Essentials

Energizing Collaboration Potential. The Collaboration Essentials presented on the opposite page are the third component of the PtC formula. The 6 Collaboration Essentials are the catalysts needed to complete the process of making PtC collaboration powerful enough to function as *Power through Collaboration.*

The Collaboration Essentials are ordered along a continuum according to the positive impact that they have on generating *Power through Collaboration.* Communication has the least impact, while Trust and Safety have the greatest impact.

The PtC Formula generates *Power through Collaboration* via a two-step process. The first step is to combine the first two components of the formula, PtC Type and PtC Motivation, to produce Collaboration Potential. As promising as this potential is, it is still just potential.

A second step needs to occur to energize potential to produce actual power. This is the energizing of Collaboration Potential by the third component of the PtC formula, the Collaboration Essentials. Without Collaboration Essentials functioning as process catalysts, Collaboration Potential created by PtC Types and Motivations remains dormant, scattered, or even clashing.

Strong Collaboration Potential alone does not guarantee *Power through Collaboration.* I frequently encounter people and organizations with very strong Collaboration Potential who still lack significant power and cannot get anything of significance done.

Sometimes people with strong Collaboration Potential cannot collaborate at all with each other. *Power through Collaboration* is nowhere to be found. Despite a favorable mix of Collaborator or Cooperator types accompanied by Shared Values and Shared Mission motivations, collaboration cannot even get off the ground. Or if it does, it quickly falls apart. Or it only produces mediocre results that are clearly out of balance with the high potential manifested.

Indeed, sometimes even people with seemingly well-matched Shared Values, Shared Mission, and Common Goals motivations cannot stand to deal with each other. Instead of collaborating, they get embroiled in conflict. Even strong Collaboration Potential from a favorable type and motivation mix requires the Collaboration Essentials in order to reliably produce *Power through Collaboration.*

Conversely and just as importantly, the Collaboration Essentials are impotent as catalysts without adequate Collaboration Potential to energize and make operational. If the Collaboration Essentials do not have any Collaboration Potential to work on, then they have nothing to activate. The three components of the PtC Formula – Collaboration Essentials, PtC Types, and PtC Motivations – all work in sync together. They are not optimally effective when deployed separately.

> When adequate levels of the 6 Collaboration Essentials energize a sufficiently favorable mix of PtC Types and Motivations, the result is *Power through Collaboration*.

In various shapes and guises the work of creating effective collaboration has typically emphasized one or another of the Collaboration Essentials process components. There are numerous programs, tools, exercises, and methods to develop and enhance the components of the Collaboration Essentials. These collaboration process components are well developed, extensively studied, and copiously utilized.

Organizing the traditional process components into the PtC Model and cumulative sequencing of the Collaboration Essentials helps to make collaboration process work more strategic. People can be more focused and effective in selecting and applying the wide variety of collaboration tools and processes.

Communication. Communication is the start of the process of trying to make collaboration work, and to take the Collaboration Essentials as far as is warranted. Hopefully all the way to Trust and Safety, because that is what makes collaboration most effective. As valuable and indispensable as Communication is for generating effective collaboration, it is worth emphasizing that Communication is just the beginning of the collaboration building process.

Communication involves putting on the table for discussion the important, sensitive, ignored, and difficult to face issues. Competing versus shared interests, goals, missions, and values all impact collaboration effectiveness and need to be discussed. Communication also involves mutual sharing of task and job related information and knowledge needed for effective performance and results.

People often attempt to achieve collaboration by emphasizing effective Communication. It may be the most common method that is utilized when people attempt to promote effective collaboration. Yet, it is weighted the lowest of the Collaboration Essentials because although Communication is essential, it is far from sufficient. Not taking into account Communication's limitations and how it best fits into an overall strategy to build collaboration has plagued many attempts to collaborate.

> Communication is just the beginning - the Collaboration Essentials' first step. Communication alone, no matter how proficient, is not the basis for collaboration, and is only adequate in the simplest of situations.

Understanding. Understanding builds upon Communication and involves developing an adequate grasp of what the task requirements, issues, interests, needs, motivations, goals, missions, and values of the parties are; to what extent such converge, diverge, or compete; and why. What is the basis for significant disagreements, and what could create greater convergence and alignment? Not only is it helpful to be clear about what affects and motivates other parties, but also oneself. Effective Communication often sharpens awareness of what is driving oneself in the collaboration endeavor.

Communication and Understanding are also needed regarding issues related to the collaboration situation at hand, including benefits and risks; how the parties are defining collaboration; and behaviors that will enhance or hinder collaboration.

When scoring Understanding as positive or negative, the criteria for a positive score is not for understanding to be supportive of the feasibility of collaboration, but that the parties have sufficient understanding of each other and their issues to make an informed decision regarding whether or not to collaborate, and how to. What is measured is the extent, quality, and accuracy of understanding.

Achieving Understanding can bridge differences and improve how well parties know each other, and improve relationships and work outcomes. But not always.

Understanding can also trigger or inflame negative reactions, such as distrust, fear, or contempt. Sometimes differences and competing interests cannot be resolved. Communication and Understanding can be effective and accurate, but suggest *Power through Collaboration* is not feasible given the parties and issues.

Sometimes the conclusion that collaboration is not feasible can be premature. Rushed or superficial processes during Communication and Understanding are susceptible to confirming early impressions, premature conclusions, and misconceptions. Or merely serving to justify what parties are already set to do.

Additionally, negative emotions and reactions can pop up early in the process of Communication and Understanding. Communicating about pivotal differing and conflicting views is integral to collaboration. Thus, disagreements and unpleasant feelings also are an expected part of collaboration. Seeing and learning things about the others that are deemed wrong or disagreeable, or finding out that one's worst fears are justified, can produce turmoil, contempt, and even repulsion.

Continued communication and persistence at working on the issues, preferably with some degree of mutual respect, is essential. As issues are delved into and nuances emerge, understanding grows and frequently ameliorates or dissolves negative reactions. Allowing the needed time for revisiting, re-evaluating, and working on genuine understanding is crucial.

> Communication and Understanding are best done with a process that does not solidify or end on the basis of first reactions.

Contrary to what is taught in most communication skills training classes, the skills needed for Communication and Understanding are very different depending upon the PtC Type you are dealing with. In general, openness, assertiveness, and tactful directness serve as optimum approaches for achieving mutual understanding with Collaborators and Cooperators. However, such popularly recommended communication approaches can be ineffective and even counterproductive when dealing with Predators and Enslavers.

Communication and Understanding are the beginning of the path to collaboration when dealing with Competitors, Cooperators, and Collaborators. Not so with Predators and Enslavers. The latter are not interested in that path, and there is no use getting on it with them unless they have improved their PtC Type.

Communication and Understanding certainly pay off with Predator and Enslaver types, but not by producing enhanced prospects for collaboration. Rather, the primary value gained is strategic information and being better able to develop an effective survival strategy with a Predator/Enslaver management plan in order to avoid being preyed upon or enslaved.

Of course, Predators and Enslavers will be doing the same. They will be doing it even if you are not. That is, using Communication and Understanding to advance their power, detect weaknesses, and gauge the best opportunities to strike. They use Communication and Understanding as an opportunity to adapt their hunting strategy to the workings of the prey. Communication can be tactically deployed to stall for time, to gain a stronger position, to wear down the prey, or distract and catch the prey off guard.

Competitor types also have a similar first reaction. That is, to use Communication and Understanding to gain the upper hand, devise a strategy to win, and defeat the other parties. At least Competitors can be worked with to some degree. Still, openness during the Communication and Understanding processes with Competitors is best paced with the extent to which they seem to be responding productively. Communication and Understanding combined with skill, good judgment, and luck, can move Competitor types toward win-win Negotiation and some degree of collaboration.

Competence. Successful Communication and Understanding do not automatically translate into wanting to collaborate with someone. Competence is a factor. Competence involves addressing the issue of whether the parties are perceived to be an asset or a liability as collaborators. Even people who are perfectly well liked, deemed undoubtedly trustworthy, and warmly regarded may not be wanted as teammates. Feeling that a person is incompetent, not up to the level of capability needed, or not contributing anything of value, sharply reduces the strength of the Collaboration Essentials. Others parties in a collaboration endeavor tend to pull back instead of engaging in collaboration with people who they feel are not sufficiently capable.

Competence requires that participants understand, agree upon, and effectively operationalize their roles, functions, and work processes. They also must be capable of performing as needed. They need to bring sufficient capability to the endeavor and add something of value that is appreciated so that they are viewed as desirable collaborators. Professional, technical, task, social, or job related capabilities need to be sufficient to garner acceptance as a participant in the collaboration enterprise. People do not need to be superstars or even highly capable, just capable enough to be accepted for whatever they can contribute. Attitude and effort can affect acceptance, sometimes more than superior capability. Expectations and demands are situation specific. In addition, specific skills related to functioning collaboratively increase the Collaboration Essentials strength.

When scoring Competence as positive or negative, the criteria for scoring in positive territory is not the degree of competence *per se*, but rather the extent to which the parties accept each other as competent enough for engaging in collaboration.

Respect. Communication and Understanding can be very effective and very accurate, yet unfavorable for collaboration. Understanding the other parties also produces a value judgment of them. Recall the saying that 'familiarity breeds contempt.' Knowing others sometimes results in a very negative reaction to and opinion of them. Sometimes for good reason.

Respect addresses the extent to which parties respect each other, the reasons for lack of respect, and what it would take to engender mutual respect. Tolerance of the parties toward each other despite their differences is essential. It goes hand in hand with collaboration, especially in a world that is becoming increasingly networked. More and more information about each other is available for open display with only few buttons or keys to push. Translating that connectivity and transparency into collaboration requires toleration and mutual acceptance. Otherwise, the result is more onerous and ubiquitous domination.

Agreements for mutual co-existence and an attitude of 'live and let live' are the minimum requirements. Greater mutual acceptance and respect increase the Collaboration Essentials strength much more than mere toleration of each other.

Much Collaboration Essentials work revolves around bridging and managing differences. Differences in point of view, strategy, values, goals, interests, personality, etcetera. When parties are at the Communication or Understanding level, differences are often viewed as problematic and troublesome. Differences are primarily viewed as an obstacle to one's own perspective or to getting one's own agenda accomplished. Significant effort is expended to minimize, bridge, neutralize, or eliminate the differences. People try to homogenize the mixture to suit their personal liking and taste.

> When Respect is achieved previously troublesome differences become viewed as advantages.

After achieving success at the Respect level, the attitude toward differences flips. The negative impact of differences becomes less troublesome or problematic. Parties cease wanting or trying to get others to be what they want or an image of themselves.

They begin to see how differences make people more interesting, and even more enjoyable. The realization dawns that different people bring something different to the table that is needed and advantageous. People no longer complain about the differences, but instead see them as an asset that enables greater success. The interplay, balancing, and integration of differences come to be viewed as a strength that leads to superior results. Consequently, the parties begin to make better use of their differences.

Respect also can extend to Predators and Enslavers, not just Collaborators and Cooperators. When communicating and seeking understanding with Predators and Enslavers, achieving a degree of respect is not unusual.

Predators and Enslavers can be awe-inspiring creatures. Many a wildly popular movie or book is based upon the captivating prowess of an infamous Predator or Enslaver. Beholding the power and capability of Predators and Enslavers often elicits respect, not unlike observing lions at feeding time in a zoo or making a kill in a game reserve.

Trust. Trust does not involve merely adopting a trusting stance with respect to the other parties. Trust work involves determining what conditions would make trust sensible, useful, and workable for the parties. And to what extent such conditions already exist, or can be created and met.

> Attempting to create trust in the absence of realistic reasons to trust is counterproductive. Working on what weakens or strengthens trust is more fruitful.

When people have trust about collaborating, Communication, Understanding, and Respect flow more naturally and easily. Less work needs to be done maintaining communication and understanding. Obviously, communication and understanding are always important, but when adequate trust exists differences and problems do not scream out to be addressed unless they are specifically related to getting the job done. Trust makes it easier to exercise toleration and stick to the important stuff. If conflict is task related, it is dealt with directly. If conflict is off task then it is accepted for what it is and only dealt with when necessary. Task and non-task conflict are less likely to become entwined and spin out of control.

Trust influences the Collaboration Essentials strength proportionally more than do the preceding Collaboration Essentials components. Even when work on Communication, Understanding, Competence, and Respect are all very successful, the conditions for trust may be missing.

Take an extreme case for example. Communication can successfully identify and delve into the relevant issues. Understanding can be clear, insightful, and thorough. Competence can be superior and easily acceptable. And Respect can be elicited by enthralling charms and enviable talents. Yet, Trust still may not be warranted because the party is a Predator or Enslaver type who is operating via Survival motivation.

Similarly, for two Competitor types who communicate directly, know each other very well, understand exactly where each stands, are highly competent and talented, and respect and like each other. Nevertheless, they cannot trust each other enough to be involved together in a collaboration enterprise.

Lack of trust puts a relatively low ceiling on potential Collaboration Essentials strength. Communication, Understanding, Competence, and Respect can all be at their maximum, yet a lack of Trust and Safety can bring Collaboration Essentials strength down to zero.

> Distrusting parties that need to cooperate are set on a collision course regarding power and control.

Lack of trust is a primary driver of conflict and power struggles. Lack of trust intensifies the need to be in control, and have control over the other parties. Lack of trust fuels the fear of being subject to control by the other parties. Distrust especially increases the sense of risk from sharing control.

Unless some workable level of trust can be developed, parties will feel that Power through Domination is their best ally and perhaps the only means of achieving their goals. Without trust parties fear being ambushed if they open up to collaboration. The more powerful and more dominant parties worry that foregoing exercising their domination capability means they will lose a window of opportunity to prevail, be set up to be taken advantage of, or become weaker. The less powerful and less dominant parties worry that collaboration lures them into closer range and increases exposure to the dominant parties' power advantage.

Progression past Trust to Safety is rare when evaluating collaboration prospects with Predators and Enslavers. Doing so requires solid reasons, but the most common reason besides lack of awareness, is desperation. With sizing up Predators and Enslavers, what can seem worthy of trust and safe one day can be the opposite the next day. Those who do move beyond Trust to Safety with regard to Predators and Enslavers almost always regret it.

Safety. Safety involves being clear about the degree of risk and exposure created by the collaboration endeavor. A sense of being at risk from collaboration weakens the Collaboration Essentials. A sense of safety provides a major boost.

The work within Safety does not involve trying to convince parties to feel safe with each other. Creating a sense of safety without valid reason can do more harm than good. As with Trust, more helpful is to determine the extent to which the parties feel safe collaborating with each other, and what weakens or strengthens a sense of safety between them. Safety work involves determining what conditions make a sense of safety reasonable, useful, and workable for the parties. And to what extent such conditions already exist, or can be created, and can be met.

Predators and Enslavers typically do not receive positive scores on Trust or Safety. All of their scores on the Collaboration Essentials may be in positive territory up to and including Respect, after which they usually stop accumulating positive scores. For most people, going any further with Predator or Enslaver types is too dangerous. What can be interesting to observe from a safe distance can be scary to engage close up. Witnessing the powerful impact of Predators and Enslavers on others may inspire awe and respect, but not a desire to be in the victim's position. When respect is mixed with fear, collaboration feels too risky. Respect without the fear is needed for collaboration.

With Predators and Enslavers there is no safety, only moments of respite or temporary periods of relatively low risk. However, desperation and the need for hope often get people to see and feel things that have little basis in reality. Prudence requires that any sense of trust or safety when engaging Predators and Enslavers should be assessed as possibly delusional.

The PtC Formula in Operation

Putting the PtC Formula into action is an extensive topic. A full discussion is beyond the scope of this book, and I already cover it in depth in the more comprehensive and advanced book *Power through Collaboration: When to Collaborate, Negotiate, or Dominate!* But, a couple of pointers are worth emphasizing here.

Understand, respect, and operate according to your own PtC Type and Motivations. To get the best out of the PtC Formula it helps to be aware of and to abide by your own type and motivations. Being fortified with such self-awareness enables you to be more strategic with respect to investing your time, energy, and other resources.

People who understand their own PtC Type and Motivations can make a more conscious and deliberate choice about who they want to engage and collaborate with at any given time. Collaboration Essentials work can be a major investment of time and energy. Engaging people with similar PtC Types and Motivations generally produces more successful Collaboration Essentials results. In particular, Collaborators and Cooperators achieve better outcomes by working together with similar types, and to the extent possible, not attempting to work collaboratively with Competitors, Enslavers, or Predators.

Although most of the time better results can be achieved from working with Collaborator and Cooperator types, sometimes Competitor types prefer to only engage other Competitor types who understand the rules of the game and want to just get things done with a minimum of what they deem to be unnecessary niceties, such as cooperation. Competitor types often view Collaborators and Cooperators as wasting time on nonessential and unproductive work processes, like the Collaboration Essentials. They want to move from deal to deal without getting bogged down. They want to just bang heads, win or lose, and then get on to the next hard-nosed round without a lot of fuss or fanfare.

Although choosing to work with people who have complementary PtC Types and PtC Motivations is most advantageous, it is not always possible. Life circumstances frequently necessitate working with various parties who have very non-complementary types and motivations. The comprehensive book *Power through Collaboration: When to Collaborate, Negotiate, or Dominate!* discusses strategy and tactics with respect to working with people who have clashing PtC Types and Motivations.

Use the PtC Formula holistically. The PtC Formula is a convenient shorthand tool that can serve as a guide in complex situations. Even when working on just one component of the PtC Formula, keep its integration with the other components in mind. Think holistically even when performing within a narrow scope. For example, even when just doing Collaboration Essentials work it is still important to keep type and motivation on the radar.

The PtC Formula generates its best results when all three components are utilized in coherence with each other, and are at sufficient levels. Without adequate Collaboration Potential from a favorable mix of PtC Types and Motivations, the Collaboration Essentials are of marginal benefit. When sufficient levels of the Collaboration Essentials energize a sufficiently favorable mix of PtC Types and Motivations, the result is *Power through Collaboration.*

Using the Collaboration Essentials process components by themselves to guide a collaboration building process, or in the absence of sufficient Collaboration Potential due to unfavorable types and motivations, is counter-productive. It significantly increases the risk of collaboration failure. However, it is a common and widespread practice that is heavily relied upon.

> Working via the Collaboration Essentials process components tends to be the primary approach to improving collaboration effectiveness. The type and motivation of the parties involved tend to be ignored, especially the PtC Types.

For decades Collaboration Essentials process components have functioned as a bastion for consultants and clients alike when working on collaboration. Training, consulting, and coaching regarding tools and processes, proscribed behaviors, and collaboration best practices have become mainstay approaches. Certainly the work can be difficult, but at least it is familiar, which makes the stress and discomfort levels more manageable. Working on the PtC Motivations is less familiar and more uncomfortable than dealing with collaboration process components.

Working on the PtC Types ratchets up the discomfort to a distressful and threatening level. In numerous situations the people issues related to types and motivations understandably are difficult, unpleasant to deal with, and acutely sensitive. Focusing on the promising potential of collaboration as well as the positive nature or potential of people is so much more gratifying than dealing with the stark reality and challenges associated with particular PtC Types.

Understand and work with the challenge of facing up to the reality of Predator and Enslaver types. When it comes to the labels that I have chosen for the PtC Types, I get completely opposite reactions. A sizable percentage of people communicate to me that they are relieved, heartened, and galvanized that I include Predators and Enslavers in the PtC classification. They welcome a model that acknowledges and addresses what they actually experience, and provides a framework to discuss the previously *undiscussable*. They deem the PtC Type labels to be an indispensable aspect of the PtC Model.

Another sizable percentage express dismay, consternation, and utter horror that I include what they deem to be such conspicuously disparaging labels in the PtC classification. For the most part they do not question the validity of the labels or the extent to which the labels reflect real-life behavior and cooperation dynamics. Rather, they feel it is inappropriate to address the issues in such unvarnished and straightforward terms. They consider such labels to be counterproductive and an obstacle to connecting with problematic types during contentious interventions.

And yet, another sizable percentage of people describe the PtC Type labels, including Predators and Enslavers, as providing a realistic picture of how people actually behave during attempted collaborations. They are relieved and encouraged by being able to discuss – albeit behind closed doors – their challenges of dealing with Predator and Enslaver types. However, their relief is encumbered by a sense of uncertainty and apprehension. Despite confiding in me their frustrations, many still are very wary about discussing such issues directly with others.

Openly discussing the more problematic types can feel improper or impolite. After all some of the people in question can be colleagues and even business associates who are worked with closely and on a regular basis. Bringing into the open their dealings with Predators and Enslavers seems like a taboo subject. It also feels extremely risky. It is the gargantuan yet proverbial elephant in the room that people cannot talk about despite being crushed breathless by its enormity.

The preference to rely on the Collaboration Essentials, in lieu of dealing with the type and motivation elephant, is very understandable. However, as valuable as the Collaboration Essentials are, they often are just not sufficient with complicated and difficult situations involving daunting obstacles to building collaboration.

> Especially in challenging situations, much of the work seemingly based on using the Collaboration Essentials to build collaboration, is actually work that implicitly requires people to change their type or motivation, or to act contrary to their type or motivation.

In such situations, the Collaboration Essentials work turns into a well-intentioned charade that skirts around and avoids acknowledging directly the work occurring to impact type and motivation. Changing or acting contrary to type and motivation, especially type, is not an easy or quick process. It requires the use of all available tools. Not being able to talk directly about type or motivation, and the lack of an enabling framework to facilitate such discussions, is a major handicap.

The PtC Model puts type and motivation clearly and prominently on the radar. It allows working on a wider range of obstacles to collaboration, thereby enhancing strategic focus and effectiveness. The PtC Types in particular offer people the option to face up to the presence of the elephant in the room. In addition, the PtC Types provide a language and concepts for tackling the sensitive and challenging issues. Thus, if working on the Collaboration Essentials or the PtC Motivations does not produce a successful result, then the PtC Types at least offers a tool and an option for dealing with that unruly elephant.

Use the PtC Formula strategically and flexibly. The PtC Formula provides options and a choice to go beyond just working with the Collaboration Essentials. Previously if work via the various Collaboration Essentials process components failed, people felt stuck and unable to proceed. With the PtC Formula, they have the option to deal with type and motivation issues that are affecting the outcome.

For example, one sign of needing to move beyond working solely via the Collaboration Essentials is when the most obvious and seemingly appealing of common goals are ignored, and provide no traction in getting the parties to work together.

Of course, the overriding consideration when operating in the field, especially under tense or stressful circumstances, is that practicality is paramount. All of the components of the PtC Formula can be used as a resource in any order that makes sense and will produce the needed results.

For example, one approach that I use to manage the discomfort of dealing with type and motivation is to deploy the PtC Formula in reverse. That is, when I work with people to develop or enhance their collaboration effectiveness I see how much mileage can be gained first via the Collaboration Essentials work. If the results from the Collaboration Essentials work do not suffice, then I engage in PtC Motivations work. If the results are still not what is needed, then I engage in PtC Types work. With this approach parties attempting to collaborate effectively need only deal with stressful issues related to PtC Types and PtC Motivations if necessary, or if they have a particular interest.

On the other hand, when I am focused on formulating a strategic vision or conducting a stakeholder analysis, I find that the PtC Formula works best when utilized according to its linear logic. The linear process helps to emphasize the value of having or developing sufficient Collaboration Potential from the mixture of PtC Types and Motivations prior to putting the Collaboration Essentials process components into action.

The preceding descriptions and discussions of the PtC Types, PtC Motivations, and Collaboration Essentials are not intended to be exhaustive or complete, but to illustrate how PtC collaboration can be operationalized in the PtC Formula. The material in this book is drawn from the primary PtC Model resource book *Power through Collaboration: When to Collaborate, Negotiate, or Dominate!* It covers the workings and implementation of the PtC Formula and Model in depth.

Collaboration is a subset of goal directed cooperative behavior in which people mutually care about achieving each other's goals and work willingly and freely to achieve each other's goals.

Power through Collaboration =

(T + M) x CE

The 5 PtC Types:

- Collaborator
- Cooperator
- Competitor
- Enslaver
- Predator

9 PtC Motivations for Cooperation:

- Survival
- External Accountability
- Internal Accountability
- Joint Defense
- Achieve Own Goals
- Common Goals
- Family & Social Bonds
- Shared Mission
- Shared Values

The 6 Collaboration Essentials:

- Communication
- Understanding
- Competence
- Respect
- Trust
- Safety

Visit: www.willisllc.com

- Take the quick and easy online PtC Collaboration Scan that is discussed in this book, and receive a chart of your results. You can also arrange a consultation regarding your PtC Collaboration Scan results.

- Check out the comprehensive and advanced book *Power through Collaboration: When to Collaborate, Negotiate, or Dominate!* that this book is drawn from.

- Obtain information about the *Power through Collaboration* workshops:

  - Introduction to the 7-Step *Power through Collaboration* Model
  - Powering Up Team Performance via the *Collaboration Essentials*
  - Advanced *Power through Collaboration* for Complex and Difficult Situations
  - Stakeholder Analysis using the PtC Model

- Join our LinkedIn discussion group to benefit from helpful, useful, and engaging exchanges regarding collaboration.

- Sign up to receive the latest news about exciting *Power through Collaboration* developments; including our forthcoming series of eBooks and the *Power through Collaboration* app.

Notes

---

[1] "Top 10 Coaches in NBA History". *NBA.com*. Retrieved April 26, 2013 from http://www.nba.com/history/top_10_coaches.html

[2] Greenspan, Alan,(October 18, 2008).Testimony given before the Government Oversight Committee of the House of Representatives.

[3] Smith, Adam (1759). *The Theory of Moral Sentiments*, page 5. London: A. Millar.

[4] Gates, Bill (2008). *A New Approach to Capitalism in the 21st Century*. World Economic Forum 2008, Davos, Switzerland. Retrieved August 10, 2010, from http://www.microsoft.com/presspass/exec/billg/speeches/2008/01-24wefdavos.mspx.

[5] Galbraith, James (2008). *The Predator State*. New York: Free Press.

[6] Drucker, Peter. The New Pluralism, *Leader to Leader*, No. 14 (Fall 1999).

[7] Boddy, Clive. The Corporate Psychopaths Theory of the Global Financial Crisis. *Journal of Business Ethics*, August 2011, Volume 102, Issue 2, pp. 255-259.

[8] Hamel, Gary and LeBarre, Polly (February 26, 2012). Reimagining Capitalism – as Principled, Patient, and Truly social. *Management Innovation EXchange*. www.managementexchange.com.

[9] http://www.ellenmacarthurfoundation.org/

[10] http://www.consciouscapitalism.org/learnmore/

[11] Sisodia, Raj (February 7, 2011). *A Better Way to Win: Profiting from Purpose*. http://www.managementexchange.com/blog/better-way-win-profiting-purpose.

[12] Keefe, Joe. "From Growth Capitalism to Sustainable Capitalism: The Next 20 Years of Sustainable Investing." *GreenMoney Journal*, Fall 2012.

[13] Declaration of Interdependence. B Lab, Inc. www.bcorporation.net

[14] Kassoy, Andrew (May 8, 2012). *Best For the World: Redefining Success in Business*. http://www.managementexchange.com/hack.

[15] www.stonyfield .com

[16] Herrera, Tilde (January 13, 2012). *Hirshberg: Why I'm Stepping Down*. Retrieved from www.greenbiz.com

[17] www.huffingtonpost.com/gary-hirshberg. (January 13, 2012).

[18] Estabrook, Barry (Jun 2 2010). Organic Growth: A Food Business Success Story. *The Atlantic*. www.theatlantic.com.

[19] Mosher, Holly (Winter 2011). GMJ Interview: Dr. Muhammad Yunus on Social Business and Microcredit. *GreenMoney Journal*, volume 20, issue 2, #82.

[20] Yunus, Muhammad (1991). Banker to the Poor: Micro-Lending and the Battle Against World Poverty. *PublicAffairs*, 1586481983.

[21] *The State of Food Insecurity in the World 2012*. Food and Agriculture Organization of the United Nations. Rome, 2012. http://www.fao.org/docrep/016/i3027e/i3027e00.htm.

[22] *U.N. chief: Hunger kills 17,000 kids daily* (November 17, 2009). CNN. http://edition.cnn.com/2009/WORLD/europe/11/17/italy.food.summit/

[23] *Global Food: Waste Not, Want Not*. January 2013. Institution of Mechanical Engineers. http://www.imeche.org/knowledge/themes/environment/global-food.

[24] *London Declaration on Neglected Tropical Diseases* (2012). www.UnitingToCombatNTDs.org.

[25] *Uniting to Combat Neglected Tropical Diseases: Translating the London Declaration into Action* (November 2012). The World Bank, Washington, D.C.

[26] *From Promises to Progress: The First Annual Report on the London Declaration on NTDs* (January 2013). www.UnitingToCombatNTDs.org.

[27] Clapper, James (September 7, 2011). How 9/11 Transformed the Intelligence Community. *Wall Street Journal*.

[28] Bamford, James. The NSA Is Building the Country's Biggest Spy Center (Watch What You Say). *Wired*, March 15, 2012. retrieved from http://www.wired.com/threatlevel/2012/03/ff_nsadatacenter/all/

[29] Herman, John D. What the Petraeus scandal says about digital spying and your e-mail. *CNN Tech,* Wed November 14, 2012. Retrieved from http://www.cnn.com/2012/11/14/tech/petraeus-email-privacy

[30] Auerbach, David. You Are What You Click: On Microtargeting. *The Nation*, March 4, 2013. http://www.thenation.com/article/172887/you-are-what-you-click-microtargeting.

[31] Smith, Gerry. Why David Petraeus' Email Troubles Should Make You Nervous. *Huff Post Tech*, 11/14/2012. Retrieved from http://www.huffingtonpost.com/2012/11/14/petraeus-scandal-protecting-private-emails_n_2129905.html.

[32] Baldor, Lolita and Cassata, Donna. General John Allen Emails To Jill Kelley Mostly Routine, Officials Say. *Huff Post Politics*, 11/16/12. Retrieved from http://www.huffingtonpost.com/2012/11/17/general-john-allen-emails_n_2151187.html.

[33] Shorrock, Tim (March 26, 2013). Obama's Crackdown on Whistleblowers. *The Nation, retrieved from http://www.thenation.com/article/173521/obamas-crackdown-whistleblowers?rel=emailNation#.*

[34] Schmidt, Eric and Cohen, Jared (2013). *The New Digital Age: Reshaping the Future of People, Nations and Business*. Alfred A. Knopf.

[35] Schmidt, Eric and Cohen, Jared. "The Dark Side of the Digital Revolution." *The Wall Street Journal*, April 19, 2013.

Made in United States
Troutdale, OR
11/03/2026

56852553R00064